AIR FRYER COOKBOOK

Healthy & Quick Recipes for Your Family

(50+ Delicious and Easy Air Fryer for Healthy)

Robert Williams

Published by Alex Howard

© **Robert Williams**

All Rights Reserved

Air Fryer Cookbook: Healthy & Quick Recipes for Your Family (50+ Delicious and Easy Air Fryer for Healthy)

ISBN 978-1-989891-81-0

All rights reserved. No part of this guide may be reproduced in any form without permission in writing from the publisher except in the case of brief quotations embodied in critical articles or reviews.

Legal & Disclaimer

The information contained in this book is not designed to replace or take the place of any form of medicine or professional medical advice. The information in this book has been provided for educational and entertainment purposes only.

The information contained in this book has been compiled from sources deemed reliable, and it is accurate to the best of the Author's knowledge; however, the Author cannot guarantee its accuracy and validity and cannot be held liable for any errors or omissions. Changes are periodically made to this book. You must consult your doctor or get professional medical advice before using any of the suggested remedies, techniques, or information in this book.

Table of Contents

Part 1 1
Introduction 2
How can you use the Air Fryer 2
Benefits of Using the Air Fryer 3
Useful Tips for Operating Your Air Fryer 4
Breakfast Recipes 6
Amazing Potato Bites with Cheese 6
Fried Eggs with Ham 8
Mac & Cheese with Topping 10
Lunch Recipes 12
Oil-Free Fried Broccoli 12
Asparagus Fries with Parmesan 14
Crunchy Jalapeno Peppers 15
Fried Tofu Cubes 16
Fried Vegetable Mix (Zucchini, Yellow Squash, and Carrots) 17
Delicious Spiced Chickpeas 18
Cauliflower Buffalo Bites 19
Classic Crispy Chicken Wings 21
Cheesy Fried Broccoli 22
Spicy Grilled Tomatoes 23
Dinner Recipes 24
Homemade Cheese Stuffed Burgers 24
Easy Cooking Pork Chop 26
Crispy Chicken Fillet with Cheese 27

Greek Meatballs with Feta	29
Crispy Air Fryer Fish	30
Amazing Fried Potatoes	31
Bacon Wrapped Chicken	32
Spicy Chicken with Rosemary	33
Stuffed Mushroom Caps	35
Fried Beef with Potatoes and Mushrooms	36
Dessert Recipes	37
Delicious Fried Bananas	37
Banana Bread	39
Cooking Measurement Conversion Chart	41
Conclusion	42
Part 2	43
Introduction	44
Benefits of the Crisplid Air Fryer	45
Vegetables Recipes	46
Crispy Ratatouille	46
Warm Quinoa And Potato Salad	48
Buttery Carrots With Pancetta	49
Braised Red Cabbage With Apples	50
Sage-Butter Spaghetti Squash	52
Parmesan Breaded Zucchini Chips	53
Spicy Sweet Potato Fries	54
Air Fried Carrots, Yellow Squash & Zucchini	55
Winter Vegetarian Frittata	58
Air Fried Kale Chips	59
Cheesy Cauliflower Fritters	59

Roasted Vegetables Salad	60
Zucchini Parmesan Chips	62
Vegetable Egg Rolls	63
Buffalo Cauliflower	64
Jumbo Stuffed Mushrooms	65
Onion Rings	66
Poultry Recipes	67
Perfect Chicken Parmesan	67
Enchilada-Braised Chicken Breasts	68
Honey-Chipotle Chicken Wings	70
Lemon and Olive Ligurian Chicken	71
Honey Soy Chicken Wings	73
Thai Green Chicken Curry	76
Chicken-Fried Steak Supreme	77
Lemon-Pepper Chicken Wings	79
Easy Turkey Breast	81
Turkey Breast	82
Paleo Turkey and Gluten-Free Gravy	83
Minty Chicken-Fried Pork Chops	84
Crispy Southern Fried Chicken	86
Tex-Mex Turkey Burgers	87
Air Fryer Turkey Breast	89
Chicken Nuggets	89
Cheesy Chicken Fritters	91
Air Fryer Chicken Parmesan	92
Ricotta and Parsley Stuffed Turkey Breasts	94
Pork Recipes	95

Pulled Pork 96
Crispy Pork Carnitas 98
Easy Pork Chops 99
Pork Chops With Applesauce 100
Spare Ribs With Wine 102
Pork Loin With Apples 103
Pork Tenderloin And Coconut Rice 105
Pork Tenderloin with Braised Apples 106
Pork Wonton Wonderful 109
Crispy Breaded Pork Chops 110
Roasted Pork Tenderloin 111
Bacon Wrapped Pork Tenderloin 112
Dijon Garlic Pork Tenderloin 113
Chinese Braised Pork Belly 114
Air Fryer Sweet and Sour Pork 115
Fried Pork Scotch Egg 117
Teriyaki Pork Rolls 118
Beef Recipes 120
Classic Pot Roast 120
Spicy Thai Beef Stir-Fry 121
Brisket With Veggies 122
Steak and Mushroom Gravy 124
Korean Braised Short Ribs 125
Meat Lovers' Pizza 127
Thai Red Beef Curry 128
Air Fryer Roast Beef 129
Beef Ribs 130

Crispy Mongolian Beef 132

Lamb Casserole 133

Swedish Meatballs 135

Barbecued Baby Back Ribs 136

Sausage And Peppers 137

Spicy Sausage And Chard Pasta Sauce 138

Ground Beef Stew 140

Lamb with Mexican Sauce 141

Pulled BBQ Beef Sandwiches 142

Air Fryer Burgers 143

Lamb And Eggplant Pasta Casserole 144

Lamb Shanks Provençal 146

Lamb Shanks With Pancetta 148

Seafood 149

Pasta with Tuna and Capers 149

Shrimp And Tomatillo Casserole 150

Fish Filets 152

Mediterranean Tuna Noodle Delight 153

Beer Potato Fish 154

Sweet And Savory Breaded Shrimp 155

Coconut Shrimp 157

Cilantro-Lime Fried Shrimp 159

Lemony Tuna 161

Grilled Soy Salmon Fillets 161

Scallops and Spring Veggies 163

Fried Calamari 164

Soy and Ginger Shrimp 164

Crispy Cheesy Fish Fingers 165
Fish Cakes With Mango Relish 166
Firecracker Shrimp 167
Sesame Seeds Coated Fish 169
Crispy Paprika Fish Fillets 169
Parmesan Shrimp 170
Fish and Chips 171
Sweet Recipes 172
Fried Peaches 172
Apple Dumplings 174
Easy Donuts 174
Cinnamon Rolls 175
Raspberry Cream Rol-Ups 176
Air Fryer Chocolate Cake 177
Chocolate Donuts 178
Fried Bananas with Chocolate Sauce 179
Apple Hand Pies 180
Chocolaty Banana Muffins 181
Blueberry Lemon Muffins 182
Sweet Cream Cheese Wontons 183
Air Fryer Cinnamon Rolls 184
Black and White Brownies 185
Baked Apple 186
Cinnamon Fried Bananas 187
HERITAGE OF FOOD: A FAMILY GATHERING 188

Part 1

Introduction

I want to start by thanking you for downloading my book. I am very pleased that thanks to my book, you will plunge into the world of quick, simple & delicious Air Fryer Recipes!

Many people love fried food but because of great taste and good smell. But they don't cook such dishes often. The reason of that is high calories and fat content in each portion of these meals.

But what will you say when I tell you about a special machine which will prepare most delicious meals you love with a minimum fat content or just without it at all? And you will enjoy cooking and taste your favorite fried meals without harm to health.

You may ask is there any way to cook French Fries, BBQ Chicken with crispy skin or any other favorite dishes without fat? Absolutely!

Only one answer is Air Fryer – the best device for you and your family! It is so easy to use that anyone can prepare delicious fried, grilled or baked meals **with 80-90% less fat** than using any pan.

Simple preparing system uses fast hot air flows around the food in a closed cooking basket inside the air fryer. You can only add one or two tablespoons of olive or vegetable oil to improve smell and taste and achieve extra crispy skin.

How can you use the Air Fryer

And finally, you decide to buy a new air fryer. You chose the model, find a place in your kitchen unpacked your purchase and get ready to cook. And after a few minutes of meditation, you realize that you do not know any recipe for the air fryer.

My Air Fryer cookbook specially issued to provide you 25 most delicious, tasty and simple recipes for your air fryer device. You can directly follow the instructions or can add some ingredients by yourself – just try and discover countless incredible recipes for your family and friends.

With the help of the air fryer, you can prepare almost any dish you love. You can grill, bake, roast, stew any ingredients in any combinations. Because of hot air circulating in the air fryer basket, all nutrients will properly and equally heat whatever size they'll have.

Only 15-30 minutes cooking after your hard working day and you will enjoy the magnificent healthy meals with minimal fat.

Just try to cook dishes using my Air Fryer Cookbook surprise your family and friends!

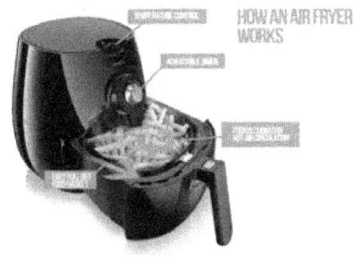

Benefits of Using the Air Fryer

Almost all of us want to eat healthy food and spend not much time for its preparation. The health benefits are main things what the air fryer has become popular for. Convenience and ease of use are secondary benefits. These and other benefits you can easily find below:

☐ Less Oil - you do not need to use more than couple tablespoon of fat while cooking dishes in the air fryer. In result, you get healthier roasted food which not soaking in unhealthy fat.

☐ Easy Cooking - it not needed to watch over your pan while frying your dinner. You just put ingredients into the fryer basket, set cooking preferences, push couple buttons and wait for the meals to get prepared.

☐ Fast Preparation - it is faster to cook in the air fryer that anywhere else. This is due to high-temperature air circulating inside the fryer basket. Hot air passes through the meals making it ready faster.

☐ Easy Cleaning - most of the air fryer details and cooking chamber are dishwasher safe. You can easily clean them either with a soapy sponge or in the dishwasher.

☐ Various Cooking - you can not only roast with the help of air fryer. You can easily bake, grill, stew in it too!

All these benefits make the air fryer number one choice among all devices in a modern kitchen. Now that you know a little more about the air fryer it is time to cook!

Useful Tips for Operating Your Air Fryer

☐ Before start using your air fryer please preheat device for 3-5 minutes. This will be enough to reach acceptable temperature for further cooking.

☐　　If you prefer cooking with using of vegetable oils you may use oil sprayers for convenient applying to food before cooking. Oils also can be used to sprinkle the fryer basket to avoid food sticking.

☐　　While cooking small items it will be useful to shake basket couple times during cooking. It will help the food such as fries, chips, chicken pieces to cook evenly.

☐　　Try not to overfill the fryer. This affects how well the air circulates around the food and also may increase cooking time and can lead to unsatisfactory results.

☐　　When you finish cooking some food fractions can stay in the fryer's basket. To loosen these pieces you may put down the basket in soapy water for 10-15 minutes before scrubbing or placing it in the dishwasher.

☐　　While cooking dishes that have high-fat content, such as pork or so, periodically remove fat from the cooking basket of your air fryer during cooking to avoid excess smoke.

☐　　When you prepare marinated or soaked in liquid dishes, dry them lightly before putting to the air fryer to avoid splattering and excess smoke.

Breakfast Recipes

Amazing Potato Bites with Cheese
Preparation time: 20 minutes, cooking time: 25 minutes.

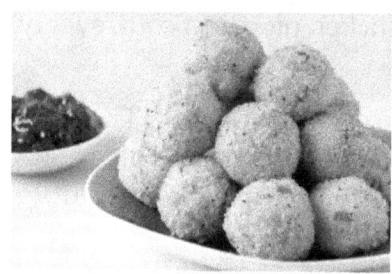

Ingredients
- 2 large Russet potatoes, peeled and cut
- ½ cup parmesan cheese, grated
- ½ cup breadcrumbs
- 2 tablespoon all-purpose flour
- ¼ teaspoon nutmeg, ground
- 2 tablespoon fresh chives, finely chopped
- 1 egg yolk
- 2 tablespoon olive oil
- ¼ teaspoon black pepper, ground
- Salt to taste

Preparation
1. In lightly salted water boil potato cubes for about 15 minutes.
2. Drain potatoes and mash them finely with the potato masher. Let them completely cool.
3. To the mashed potato add egg yolk, grated cheese, chives, and flour.
4. Season the mixture with ground pepper, nutmeg, and salt.

5. Make 1 ½ inch balls and place them in the flour and then to the breadcrumbs.
6. Preheat the Air Fryer to 370-390°F
7. Carefully place handmade potato rolls to the Air Fryer basket and cook for about 10 minutes, until they become golden brown.
8. Serve either warm or cold and enjoy!

Fried Eggs with Ham
Preparation time: 5 minutes, cooking time: 10-15 minutes.

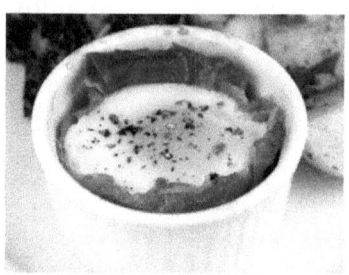

Ingredients
- 4 large eggs
- 2 oz (nearly 2 thin slices) ham
- 2 teaspoon butter
- 2 tablespoon heavy cream
- 3 tablespoon parmesan cheese, grated
- 2 teaspoon fresh chives, chopped
- A pinch of smoked paprika
- Salt and ground black pepper to taste

Preparation
1. Grease the pie pan with butter and line the bottom with ham slices. Make the bottom and sides of the pie pan completely covered with ham.
2. In a small bowl beat 1 egg, add heavy cream, a pinch of salt and 1/8 teaspoon ground pepper. Whisk to combine.
3. Pour this egg mixture over the ham and beat remaining 3 eggs over top.
4. Season with salt and ground pepper, sprinkle with parmesan cheese.

5. Preheat the Air Fryer to 320-350°F
6. Place the pie pan into the cooking basket and cook for 12 minutes.
7. When finished, remove fried eggs from the pie pan with the help of spatula and transfer to the plate. Season with smoked paprika and chopped chives.

Mac & Cheese with Topping
Preparation time: 20 minutes, cooking time: 5 minutes.

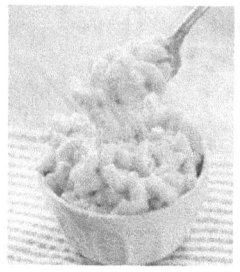

Ingredients
- 3 cups macaroni
- 15 pcs Ritz biscuits
- 2 oz gruyere cheese, grated
- 2 oz butter
- 2 tablespoon plain flour
- 16 oz milk
- 1 clove garlic, minced
- 1 cup pizza cheese mix (Mozzarella, Parmesan, Cheddar)

Preparation
1. Crush Ritz biscuits, mix with gruyere cheese and set aside.
2. Cook macaroni until almost ready, drained and also set aside.
3. Melt the butter in the separate bowl on the small fire and fry the garlic until fragrant. Add plain flour. Add milk and stir until mixture thickens and looks like a creamy soup. Add remained gruyere cheese and let it melt in the sauce.
4. Bring this sauce to a simmer and switch off the fire. Add macaroni into the mixture and combine well.
5. Dish into individual ceramic bowls.
6. Spoon with Ritz biscuits mixture over macaroni. Top with pizza cheese mix.
7. Preheat the air fryer to 350°F

8. Place ceramic bowls into the Air Fryer and cook for 5 minutes or until pizza cheese mix becomes golden.
9. Serve warm and enjoy.

Lunch Recipes

Oil-Free Fried Broccoli
Preparation time: 40 minutes, cooking time: 10 minutes.

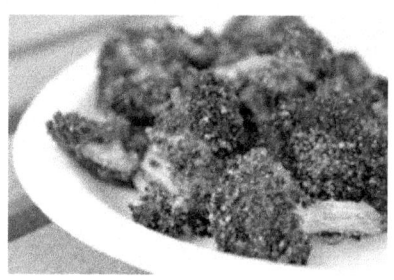

Ingredients
- 1 pound broccoli
- 1 tablespoon chickpea flour
- For marinade
- 1 tablespoon yogurt
- ¼ teaspoon turmeric powder
- ½ teaspoon chili powder
- ½ teaspoon Chat Masala
- 1 pinch salt

Preparation
1. Cut broccoli into small florets. Dip florets in the large bowl of water and 2 tablespoons salt for 20-30 minutes to remove different insects.
2. Remove from the salty water, drain well and remove extra water using paper towels.
3. In the bowl mix all ingredients for the marinade: yogurt, turmeric powder, chili powder, Chat Masala.
4. Toss the broccoli florets in the marinade and set aside in the refrigerator for 15-20 minutes.

5. Preheat the Air Fryer to 370-390°F
6. Place marinated broccoli florets into the Fryer basket and cook for 10 minutes.
7. Shake once during cooking. Prepare until become golden and crispy.
8. Serve warm and enjoy.

Asparagus Fries with Parmesan
Preparation time: 10 minutes, cooking time: 10 minutes.

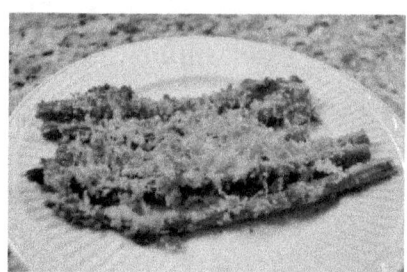

Ingredients
- 15-20 asparagus spears
- ½ cup flour
- 1 egg, beaten
- ½ cup whole grain breadcrumbs
- ½ cup parmesan cheese, grated

Preparation
1. Dip the asparagus spears in the flour and shake off the excess.
2. Then dip them into the beaten egg and then into the breadcrumbs.
3. Preheat the Air Fryer to 390°F
4. Place coated asparagus spears into the Air Fryer basket and cook for 10 minutes.
5. Remove them and sprinkle with grated parmesan cheese on the top.
6. Cook for another 3-5 minutes until cheese becomes golden brown.

Crunchy Jalapeno Peppers

Preparation time: 20 minutes, cooking time: 10 minutes.

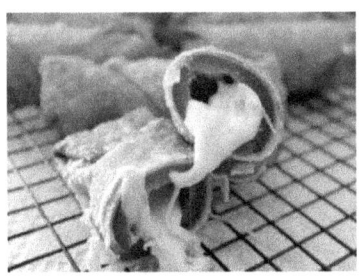

Ingredients

- 2-3 jalapeno peppers, sliced
- 1 oz cheddar cheese
- 1 spring roll wrapper
- 1 tablespoon Egg Beaters

Preparation

1. Firstly prepare peppers: cut stem end off, slice lengthwise, trim out all seeds and inner core.
2. Cut cheese into ½ oz strips.
3. Peel off a sheet of spring roll wrapper and cut in half. Cover each half with a half tablespoon of liquid egg mixture.
4. Place a half of jalapeno pepper in one corner of the spring roll wrapper half (egg-brushed side up), then place a strip of cheese and then another half of jalapeno.
5. Roll the pepper and cheese tightly in the spring roll wrapper on the diagonal.
6. Check all sides and glue any loose edges with egg mixture.
7. Preheat the Air Fryer to 370°F
8. Lightly spray each wrapping with cooking spray and put them into the Fryer. Cook for about 10 minutes until they become brown.

9. Serve hot or warm.

Fried Tofu Cubes
Preparation Time: 10 minutes, cooking time: 20 minutes.

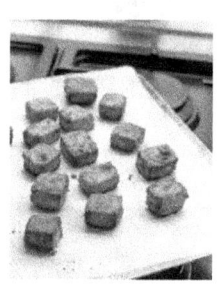

Ingredients
- 12 oz Low-Fat Tofu
- 2 tablespoon soy sauce
- 2 tablespoon fish sauce
- 1 teaspoon sesame or olive oil
- 1 teaspoon Maggi

Preparation
1. Cut tofu into 1 inch cubes, place in the medium bowl and set aside.
2. In the large bowl combine all ingredients and make a marinade.
3. Dip tofu to the marinade for at least 20-30 minutes.
4. Preheat the Air Fryer to 370°F
5. Put marinated tofu cubes and cook for 15 minutes. If you want extra crispy cubes, cook for 20-25 minutes.
6. Serve and enjoy!

Fried Vegetable Mix (Zucchini, Yellow Squash, and Carrots)

Preparation time: 10 minutes, cooking time: 35 minutes.

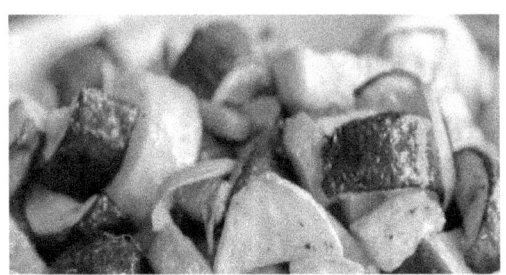

Ingredients
- ½ pound carrots, peeled
- 1 pound zucchini
- 1 pound yellow squash
- 2-3 tablespoon olive oil
- 1 teaspoon salt
- ½ teaspoon ground white pepper
- 1 tablespoon tarragon leaves, chopped

Preparation
1. Cut carrots into 1-inch cubes, mix with 1 tablespoon of olive oil and stir to combine.
2. Preheat the Air Fryer to 390°F
3. Place carrots to the Air Fryer and cook for 5 minutes.
4. While carrots cook, prepare other vegetables. Trim stem and root ends from zucchini and cut into ¾-inch half

moons. Also, trim stem and root end from yellow squash and cut into ¾-inch half moons.
5. Place vegetables into large mixing bowl and sprinkle with the remaining olive oil, season with white pepper and salt. Coat all vegetables evenly.
6. Once the time in the Air Fryer goes off, add there zucchini and yellow squash.
7. Cook for another 30 minutes, mixing couple time through the cooking process.
8. When vegetables prepared, remove them and sprinkle with tarragon.
9. Serve warm and enjoy.

Delicious Spiced Chickpeas
Preparation time: 5 minutes, cooking time: 20 minutes.

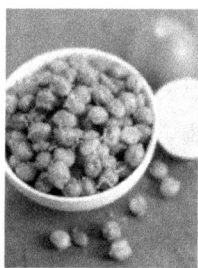

Ingredients
- 1 can (15 oz) chickpeas, rinsed & drained
- 1 tablespoon olive oil
- 1 teaspoon paprika
- ½ tablespoon cumin
- 1 teaspoon salt

- A pinch of cayenne pepper

Preparation
1. In the large bowl mix together the chickpeas, olive oil, paprika, cumin, salt and cayenne pepper.
2. Preheat the Air Fryer to 370-390°F
3. Divide chickpeas mixture in batches and place into the Air Fryer. Cook for 8-10 minutes and shake the basket in the middle of cooking.
4. Transfer prepared chickpeas to a bowl and season with salt to taste.

Cauliflower Buffalo Bites
Preparation time: 5 minutes, cooking time: 20 minutes.

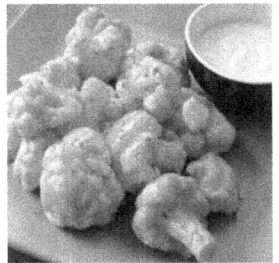

Ingredients
- 1 large head cauliflower, cut into florets
- 1 tablespoon olive oil
- 2 teaspoon garlic powder
- ½ cup Buffalo Style sauce or other hot sauce for your choice
- 1 tablespoon melted butter
- ¼ teaspoon salt
- ¼ teaspoon ground pepper

Preparation
1. Cut cauliflower into bite-sized florets.

2. Place cauliflower florets into large plastic bag add olive oil, garlic powder, salt, and pepper. Close bag and toss ingredients and make sure all florets coated.
3. Preheat the Air Fryer to 400°F
4. Place coated florets to the cooking basket and cook for 15 minutes, turning once during cooking.
5. Remove cauliflower from the fryer.
6. Melt the butter and add the hot sauce. Toss florets and cover all of them with this mixture.
7. Return to the Air Fryer and cook for another 5 minutes.
8. Serve warm with any sauce you prefer, for example, blue cheese dip or sour cream.

Classic Crispy Chicken Wings
Preparation time: 5 minutes, cooking time: 35 minutes.

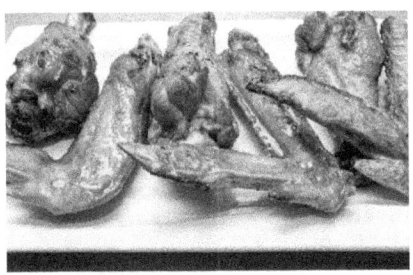

Ingredients
- 1 pound chicken wings
- 2 tablespoon Provencal herbs
- 1 teaspoon black ground pepper
- Salt to taste

Preparation
1. In the large mixing bowl add chicken wings and coat them evenly with salt, ground pepper, and Provencal herbs. Mix with hands.
2. Preheat the Air Fryer to 370-390°F
3. Spray the cooking basket with a nonstick coating.
4. Place coated wings into the Air Fryer basket and cook for 15-20 minutes. Shake couple times during cooking.
5. Maybe it will need to repeat the operation until all wings become golden.
6. Serve with your favorite dipping sauce (I prefer BBQ but Buffalo, Ranch or Blue Cheese is also OK). Enjoy!

Cheesy Fried Broccoli
Preparation time: 10-12 minutes, cooking time: 25 minutes.

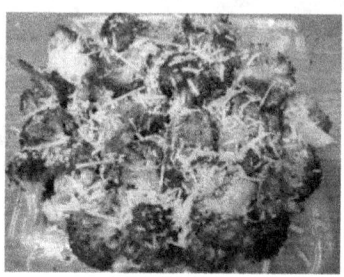

Ingredients
- 2 pounds broccoli, cut into florets
- 2 tablespoon olive oil
- 1/3 cup Kalamata olives, pitted and halved
- ½ teaspoon ground black pepper
- 2 teaspoon lemon zest, grated
- 4-6 slices parmesan cheese
- A pinch of salt

Preparation
1. Cook broccoli florets into salted water. Remove from the water drain well and toss with olive oil, salt, and pepper.
2. Preheat the Air Fryer to 370-390°F
3. Place oiled broccoli into the Fryer and cook for 15 minutes, shaking couple times during frying.
4. When the timer goes off, remove cooked broccoli and transfer to the serving bowl.
5. Toss with halved olives, lemon zest, and parmesan slices and serve.

Spicy Grilled Tomatoes
Preparation time: 5 minutes, cooking time: 20 minutes.

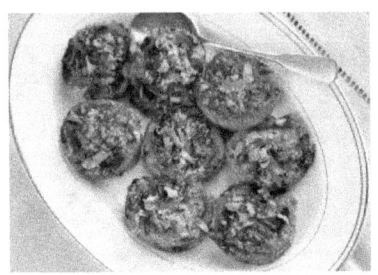

Ingredients
- 2 medium tomatoes, sliced
- Herbs you like (I prefer Provencal herbs but it can be parsley, oregano, basil, thyme, rosemary or something else)
- Ground pepper and salt to taste
- 1 tablespoon olive oil or cooking spray

Preparation
1. Wash tomatoes, dry them with paper kitchen towels.
2. Cut them in half. Turn halves cut side up. Sprinkle tops with olive oil or cooking spray. Season with ground pepper and herbs dried or fresh.
3. Set your Air Fryer to 320 °F (without preheating), place tomato halves and cook for 20 minutes. Depending on tomatoes size, how many halves you prepare and your personal preference preparation time can vary.

Tip: you can serve grilled tomatoes piping hot, room temperature or chilled.

Dinner Recipes

Homemade Cheese Stuffed Burgers
Preparation time: 10 minutes, cooking time: 20 minutes.

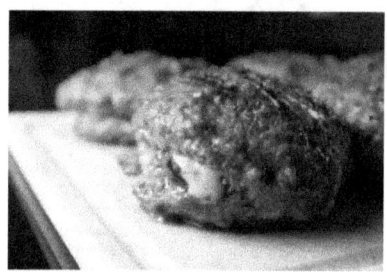

Ingredients
- 1 pound finely ground beef
- 2 oz cheddar cheese
- Salt and ground pepper to taste

Preparation
1. Take the large mixing bowl and put minced beef. Break it up and season with salt and black pepper.
2. Divide the mince into 4 balls.
3. Cut the cheese into 4 equal pieces.
4. Take half mince from one of the balls and form it into a circle about 2.5 inch wide.
5. Push a piece of the cheese into the center of the mince ball.
6. From the remaining half of mince make the circle with the same width and put on the top. Carefully join the base with cheese and the top and then gently form the burger with your hands.
7. Preheat the Air Fryer to 370°F

8. Cook burgers in the Air Fryer for about 15-20 minutes until they become ready turning halfway through the cooking time.

Easy Cooking Pork Chop
Preparation time: 15 minutes, cooking time: 15 minutes.

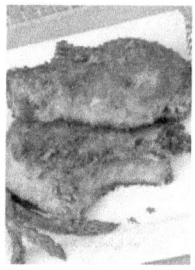

Ingredients
- 2 middle pieces pork chop
- 1 tablespoon plain flour
- 1 egg, beaten
- 2 tablespoon olive oil
- 3 tablespoon breadcrumbs
- Salt and ground pepper for seasoning

Preparation
1. Season pork chop with salt and ground pepper from both sides.
2. In three different bowls place plain flour, beaten egg, and breadcrumbs.
3. Coat each pork chop from both sides first with flour then with egg and with breadcrumbs.
4. Preheat the Air Fryer to 380°F
5. Place coated pork chops into the Fryer and cook for 10 minutes from one side and 5 minutes from another side.
6. Serve with cooked rice and mashed potatoes.

Crispy Chicken Fillet with Cheese

Preparation time: 10 minutes, cooking time: 15 minutes.

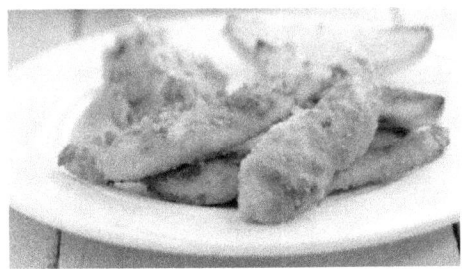

Ingredients
- 2 pounds chicken tenders (you may also choose chicken legs, boneless and skinless)
- ½ cup parmesan cheese
- 1 cup Panko breadcrumbs
- 1 oz butter, melted
- 1 egg
- 1 teaspoon garlic powder
- 1 teaspoon Italian herbs

Preparation
1. In the large bowl mix beaten egg, melted butter, garlic powder and, Italian herbs.
2. Marinate chicken tenders into the mixture for at least 30 minutes.
3. I another bowl mix Panko breadcrumbs with parmesan cheese.
4. Cover chicken meat with breadcrumb mixture and leave for 5 minutes.
5. Preheat the Air Fryer to 350°F

6. Place chicken tenders into the fryer and cook for 5-6 minutes. Then flip to another side and cook for another 3-5 minutes, until chicken becomes golden and ready.
7. Serve immediately with dipping sauce you prefer.

Greek Meatballs with Feta

Preparation time: 10 minutes, cooking time: 10 minutes.

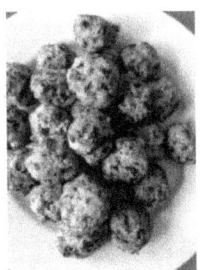

Ingredients
- ½ pound ground beef
- 1 slice white bread, crumbled
- ¼ cup feta cheese, crumbled
- 1 tablespoon fresh oregano, chopped
- 1 tablespoon fresh parsley, chopped
- ½ teaspoon ground black pepper
- A pinch of salt

Preparation
1. In the large mixing bowl combine ground beef, breadcrumbs, fresh herbs, ground pepper and salt. Mix well to receive smooth paste.
2. Divide the mixture into 8-10 equal pieces.
3. Wet your hands and roll meatballs.
4. Preheat the Air Fryer to 370-390°F
5. Place meatballs into the Fryer and cook for 8-10 minutes, depending on the size of your meatballs.
6. Serve with rice or pasta.

Crispy Air Fryer Fish
Preparation time: 10 minutes, cooking time: 12-15 minutes.

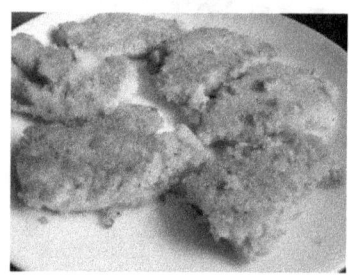

Ingredients
- 4 fish fillets (as you desired)
- 1 egg, whisked
- 3 oz breadcrumbs
- 2 tablespoon olive oil
- 1 lemon to serve

Preparation
1. In the small bowl whisk one egg and set aside.
2. In another bowl mix oil and breadcrumbs. Stir to combine until becomes loose and crumbly.
3. Preheat the Air Fryer to 360°F
4. Dip prepared fish fillets into whisked egg and then into the breadcrumbs mixture. Make sure that fillets fully breaded.
5. Lay covered fillets in the Air Fryer and cook for 12-15 minutes. Cooking time may vary depending on the fillets thickness.
6. Serve with sliced lemon and enjoy.

Amazing Fried Potatoes
Preparation time: 15 minutes, cooking time: 1 hour 50 minutes.

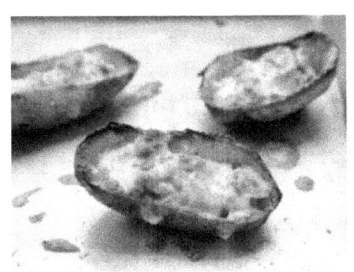

Ingredients
- 2 (15oz) potatoes
- 2 stripes bacon, chopped
- 1/3 cup cheddar cheese
- 1 tablespoon green onion, chopped
- 1 tablespoon butter
- 1 teaspoon olive oil
- A pinch of salt
- Ground black pepper to taste

Preparation
1. Preheat the Air Fryer to 370-390°F
2. Rub potatoes with olive oil and cook in the Fryer for 30-50 minutes until it becomes fork tender. Remove potatoes from the Air Fryer and set aside to cool.
3. While potatoes cooks, chop bacon stripes into ½ inch pieces, put in a sauté pan and cook until it becomes crispy

and golden, for nearly 10 minutes. Remove cooked bacon and set aside.
4. Take chilled potatoes and cut it in half lengthwise. Using a spoon scoop out potato pulp leaving about 1/4 inch border of potato pulp next to the skin.
5. Add cooked bacon and its fat to the potato pulp, ¼ cup of shredded cheese, 1 ½ teaspoon of green onion, butter, salt, and pepper. Stir to combine.
6. Divide the mixture between potato skins and fill them. Sprinkle potato halves with the remaining cheese.
7. Place potatoes to the Air Fryer basket side by side and cook at 390°F for about 15-20 minutes until cheese melted and becomes golden brown.
8. Once cooked replace potatoes from the Fryer and sprinkle with the remaining green onion.
9. Serve warm.

Bacon Wrapped Chicken
Preparation time: 10 minutes, cooking time: 15 minutes.

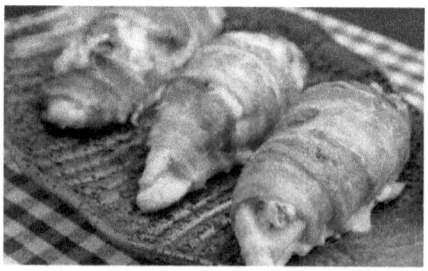

Ingredients
- 1 pound chicken tender, skinless and boneless
- 4-6 bacon stripes
- 4 tablespoon brown sugar
- ½ teaspoon chili powder

Preparation
1. In the large bowl mix brown sugar and chili powder.
2. Cut chicken tenders into 2-inch pieces.
3. Wrap chicken pieces into bacon strips and toss with sugar mixture.
4. Preheat the Air Fryer to 390-400°F
5. Place wrapped chicken into the Fryer and cook for about 10-15 minutes depending on the size of the chicken.
6. Replace the meal from the cooking basket and enjoy crispy bacon and tender, juicy chicken. You may use dipping sauce you prefer.

Spicy Chicken with Rosemary
Preparation time: 15 minutes, cooking time: 30 minutes.

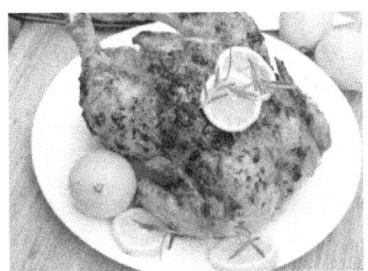

Ingredients
- 1 whole chicken (4-5 pounds)
- 2 cups potatoes, diced
- ½ large onion, diced
- 3 garlic cloves, minced

- 1 ½ teaspoon black pepper
- 1 ½ teaspoon dried thyme
- 1 ½ teaspoon dried rosemary
- 1 ½ teaspoon dried paprika
- 2 teaspoon olive oil
- 1 ½ teaspoon salt
- Fresh rosemary and sliced lemon for decoration

Preparation
1. Clean the chicken inside. Do not cut.
2. Marinate the chicken with 1 teaspoon salt and 1 teaspoon black pepper. Set aside for 20-30 minutes.
3. In the large bowl mix diced potato and diced onion with ½ teaspoon salt and pepper, 1 teaspoon paprika, thyme, and rosemary.
4. In another small bowl mix olive oil, ½ teaspoon dried, ½ dried thyme, minced garlic.
5. Preheat the Air Fryer to 400°F
6. Stuff vegetable mixture into the chicken, and cover it with garlic sauce.
7. Wrap stuffed chicken with foil and cook in the Air Fryer for 30 minutes until chicken will become golden and ready.
8. Replace the chicken to the serving plate take potatoes and onion out of the chicken.
9. Decorate with lemon and fresh rosemary.

Stuffed Mushroom Caps
Preparation time: 10 minutes, cooking time: 5 minutes.

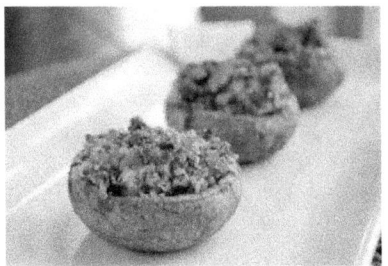

Ingredients
- 10 mushrooms
- 4 bacon slices, cut
- ¼ middle onion, diced
- ½ cup cheese, grated
- Ground black pepper and salt to taste

Preparation
1. Wash mushrooms, drain well and remove stems.
2. In the middle bowl combine bacon, cut into ½ inch pieces, diced onion and grated cheese.
3. Season mushroom caps with salt and pepper.
4. Put bacon mixture to the seasoned mushroom caps.
5. Preheat the Air Fryer to 380°F
6. Place mushrooms into the Fryer and cook for 5 minutes until cheese melted.
7. Serve and enjoy.

Fried Beef with Potatoes and Mushrooms
Preparation time: 20 minutes, cooking time: 15 minutes.

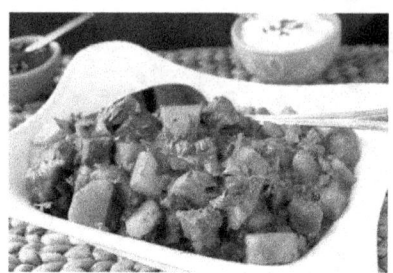

Ingredients
1. 1 pound beef steak
2. 1 medium onion, sliced
3. 8 oz mushrooms, sliced
4. ½ pound potatoes, diced
5. Sauce you prefer (Barbecue or Teriyaki)
6. Salt and black pepper for seasoning

Preparation
1. Wash vegetables, chop onion and mushrooms, dice potatoes.
2. Sprinkle them with salt and pepper.
3. Cut beef steak into 1 inch pieces.
4. In the large mixing bowl combine onion, potatoes, mushrooms and beef. Marinate with sauce and set aside for 15-20 minutes.
5. Preheat the Air Fryer to 350-370°F
6. Put meat and vegetables into the Fryer and cook for 15 minutes.
7. After cooking replace the meal to the serving plate and sprinkle with fresh chopped parsley.

Dessert Recipes

Delicious Fried Bananas
Preparation time: 3 minutes, cooking time: 8 minutes.

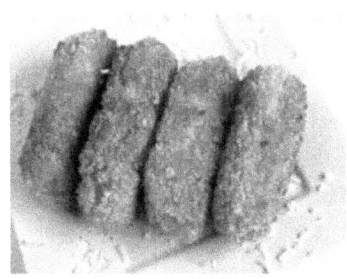

Ingredients
- 2 large bananas
- ½ cup plain flour
- 2 eggs, whisked
- ¾ cup breadcrumbs
- ½ cup cinnamon sugar
- 1 tablespoon olive oil
- A pinch of salt

Preparation
1. Take 4 bowls and place separately: flour with salt, whisked eggs, breadcrumbs, and cinnamon sugar.
2. Peel bananas and cut them into thirds. Evenly cover bananas with the flour, then with eggs, and finally with breadcrumbs.
3. Preheat the Air Fryer to 360°F
4. Sprinkle covered bananas with olive oil and put into the Air Fryer. Cook for 4-5 minutes, and then make a shake to move bananas. Cook for another 4-5 minutes.

5. Remove the bananas and through then directly into the cinnamon sugar.
6. Get them cool for a minute and eat!

Banana Bread
Preparation time: 15 minutes, cooking time: 1 hour 25 minutes.

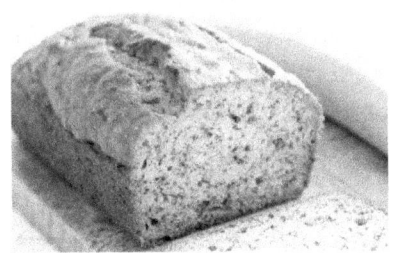

Ingredients
- ½ ripe banana, peeled
- 2 eggs
- 4 tablespoon unsalted butter, plus 2 teaspoons
- ¾ cup flour, plus some more for dusting the loaf pan
- 1/3 cup pecans, lightly toasted and chopped
- ¼ cup brown sugar
- ¼ cup granulated sugar
- ¾ teaspoon vanilla extract
- 1 teaspoon ground cinnamon
- ¼ teaspoon ground nutmeg
- A pinch of salt
- ¼ teaspoon baking soda
- 1/8 teaspoon baking powder

Preparation
1. Grease the loaf pan with 2 teaspoons of butter and dust the inner side with flour. Set aside.
2. In a mixing bowl place a half of the banana and brown sugar. Combine using the back of the spoon.

3. Add eggs, granulated sugar, vanilla extract, cinnamon, nutmeg, and salt and whisk thoroughly to combine.
4. Sift in flour, baking soda and baking powder. Stir to combine.
5. Pour the batter into the prepared loaf pan and sprinkle with pecans.
6. Preheat the Air Fryer to 310-330°F
7. Place the loaf pan into the Fryer and cook for 30 minutes.
8. Then check the bread with a cake tester or wooden skewer and cook more until tester will come out clean.
9. Remove from the loaf pan, cut into slices and serve with honey or another topping.

Cooking Measurement Conversion Chart

Liquid Measures

1 gal = 4 qt = 8 pt = 16 cups = 128 fl oz
½ gal = 2 qt = 4 pt = 8 cups = 64 fl oz
¼ gal = 1 qt = 2 pt = 4 cups = 32 fl oz
½ qt = 1 pt = 2 cups = 16 fl oz
¼ qt = ½ pt = 1 cup = 8 fl oz

Dry Measures

1 cup = 16 Tbsp = 48 tsp = 250ml
¾ cup = 12 Tbsp = 36 tsp = 175ml
⅔ cup = 10 ⅔ Tbsp = 32 tsp = 150ml
½ cup = 8 Tbsp = 24 tsp = 125ml
⅓ cup = 5 ⅓ Tbsp = 16 tsp = 75ml
¼ cup = 4 Tbsp = 12 tsp = 50ml
⅛ cup = 2 Tbsp = 6 tsp = 30ml
1 Tbsp = 3 tsp = 15ml

Dash or Pinch or Speck = less than ⅛ tsp

Quickies

1 fl oz = 30 ml
1 oz = 28.35 g
1 lb = 16 oz (454 g)
1 kg = 2.2 lb
1 quart = 2 pints

U.S.	Canadian
¼ tsp	1.25 mL
½ tsp	2.5 mL
1 tsp	5 mL
1 Tbl	15 mL
¼ cup	50 mL
⅓ cup	75 mL
½ cup	125 mL
⅔ cup	150 mL
¾ cup	175 mL
1 cup	250 mL
1 quart	1 liter

Recipe Abbreviations

Cup = c or C
Fluid = fl
Gallon = gal
Ounce = oz
Package = pkg
Pint = pt
Pound = lb or #
Quart = qt
Square = sq
Tablespoon = T or Tbl
  or TBSP or TBS
Teaspoon = t or tsp

Fahrenheit (°F) to Celcius (°C)
°C = (°F - 32) x 5/9

32 °F	0 °C
40 °F	4 °C
140 °F	60 °C
150 °F	65 °C
160 °F	70 °C
225 °F	107 °C
250 °F	121 °C
275 °F	135 °C
300 °F	150 °C
325 °F	165 °C
350 °F	177 °C
375 °F	190 °C
400 °F	205 °C
425 °F	220 °C
450 °F	230 °C
475 °F	245 °C
500 °F	260 °C

OVEN TEMPERATURES

WARMING: 200 °F
VERY SLOW: 250 °F - 275 °F
SLOW: 300 °F - 325 °F
MODERATE: 350 °F - 375 °F
HOT: 400 °F - 425 °F
VERY HOT: 450 °F - 475 °F

*Some measurements were rounded

Conclusion

I hope this book has helped you realize how essential role played the air fryer in preparing healthy dishes. And if you practice a healthy lifestyle, using the air fryer at home is the right choice.

As you understand from this cookbook there are a lot of dishes you can cook with the help of the air fryer. But you always can create your own dishes, combining your favorite ingredients.

Enjoy healthy fried food without oil prepared at home.

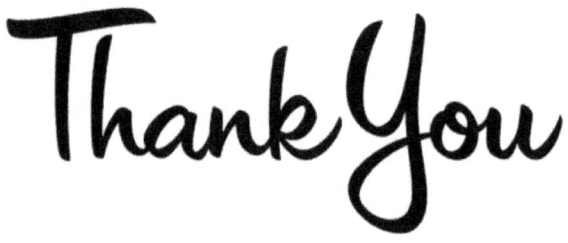

Part 2

Introduction

The Crisplid for Pressure Cooker - Turns your Pressure Cooker into an Air Fryer, and is an easy way to cook delicious healthy meals. Rather than cooking the food in oil and hot fat that may affect your health, the machine uses rapid hot air to circulate around and cook meals. This allows the outside of your food to be crispy and also makes sure that the inside layers are cooked through.

Crisplid allows us to cook almost everything and a lot of dishes. We can use the Crisplid for cooking Meat, vegetables, poultry, fruit, fish, and a wide variety of desserts. It is possible to prepare your entire meals, starting from appetizers to main courses as well as desserts. Not to mention, Crisplid also allows homemade preserves or even delicious sweets and cakes.

How Does Crisplid Works?
The technology of the Crisplid Air Fryer is very simple. Fried foods get their crunchy texture because hot oil heats foods quickly and evenly on their surface. Oil is an excellent heat conductor, which helps with fast and simultaneous cooking across all of the ingredients. For decades cooks have used convection ovens to try to mimic the effects of frying or to cook the whole surface of the food. But the air never circulates quickly enough to achieve that delicious surface crisp we all love in fried foods.

With this mechanism, the air is circulated on high degrees, up to 200° C, to "air fry" any food such as fish, chicken or chips, etc. This technology has changed the whole idea of cooking by reducing the fat up to 80% compared to old-fashioned deep fat frying.

The Crisplid Air Fryer cooking releases the heat through a heating element that cooks the food in a healthier and more appropriate way. There's also an exhaust fan right above the cooking chamber, which provides the food required airflow. This way, food is cooked with constant heated air. This leads to the same heating temperature reaching every single part of the food that is being cooked. So, this is only grill and the exhaust fan that is helping the Crisplid Air Fryer to boost air at a constantly high speed in order to cook healthy food with less fat.

The internal pressure increases the temperature that will then be controlled by the exhaust system. Exhaust fan also releases extra filtered air to cook the food in a much healthier way. The Crisplid Air Fryer has no odor at all, and it is absolutely harmless, making it user and environment-friendly.

Enjoy!

Benefits of the Crisplid Air Fryer

- Converts a Pressure Cooker in an Air Fryer. (fits 6 and 8 quart stainless steel inner pots)
- Healthier, oil-free meals
- It eliminates cooking odors through internal air filters
- Makes cleaning easier due to lack of oil grease
- Crisplid Air Fryer is able to bake, grill, roast and fry providing more options
- A safer method of cooking compared to deep frying with exposed hot oil
- Has the ability to set and leave as most models and it includes a digital timer

The Crisplid Air Fryer is an all-in-one that allows cooking to be easy and quick. It also leads to a lot of possibilities once you get to know it. Once you learn the basics and become familiar with your Crisplid Air Fryer, you can feel free to experiment and modify the recipes in the way you prefer. You can prepare a wide number of dishes with the Crisplid Air Fryer and you can adapt your favorite stove-top dish so it becomes Air Fryer–friendly. It all boils down to variety and lots of options, right?
Cooking perfect and delicious as well as healthy meals has never been easier. You can see how this recipe collection proves itself.

Enjoy!

Vegetables Recipes

Crispy Ratatouille

PREP: 5 MINUTES • PRESSURE: 4 MINUTES • BROIL: 5 MINUTES • TOTAL: 14 MINUTES • PRESSURE LEVEL: HIGH • RELEASE: QUICK
SERVES 4

Ingredients
Kosher salt, for salting and seasoning
1 small eggplant, peeled and sliced ½ inch thick
1 medium zucchini, sliced ½ inch thick
2 tablespoons olive oil
1 cup chopped onion
3 garlic cloves, minced or pressed
1 small green bell pepper, cut into ½-inch chunks (about 1 cup)

1 small red bell pepper, cut into ½-inch chunks (about 1 cup)
1 rib celery, sliced (about 1 cup)
1 (14.5-ounce) can diced tomatoes, undrained
¼ cup water
½ teaspoon dried oregano
¼ teaspoon freshly ground black pepper
2 tablespoons minced fresh basil
¼ cup pitted green or black olives (optional)

Directions
1.   Preparing the Ingredients. Place a rack on a baking sheet. With kosher salt, very liberally salt one side of the eggplant and zucchini slices, and place them, salted-side down, on the rack. Salt the other side. Let the slices sit for 15 to 20 minutes, or until they start to exude water (you'll see it beading up on the surface of the slices and dripping into the sheet pan). Rinse the slices, and blot them dry. Cut the zucchini slices into quarters and the eggplant slices into eighths.
Turn the Multicooker to "Sauté", heat the olive oil until it shimmers and flows like water. Add the onion and garlic, and sprinkle with a pinch or two of kosher salt. Cook for about 3 minutes, stirring until the onions just begin to brown.
Add the eggplant, zucchini, green bell pepper, red bell pepper, celery, and tomatoes with their juice, water, and oregano.
2.   High pressure for 4 minutes. Lock the lid on the Multicooker and then cook for 4 minutes. To get 4-minutes cook time, press "Pressure" button and use the Time Adjustment button to adjust the cook time to 4 minutes.
3.   Pressure Release. Use the quick-release method.
4.   Finish the dish. Unlock and remove the lid. Close the CRISPING LID. Select BROIL, and set the time to 5 minutes. Select START/STOP to begin. Cook until top is browned.
Stir in the pepper, basil, and olives (if using). Taste, adjust the seasoning as needed, and serve.

While this vegetable dish is usually served on its own, it's great tossed with cooked pasta or served over polenta.

PER SERVING: CALORIES: 149; FAT: 8G; SODIUM: 55MG; CARBOHYDRATES: 20G; FIBER: 8G; PROTEIN: 4G

Warm Quinoa And Potato Salad

PREP: 5 MINUTES • PRESSURE: 10 MINUTES • BROIL: 5 MINUTES • TOTAL: 20 MINUTES • PRESSURE LEVEL: HIGH • RELEASE: QUICK
SERVES 6

Ingredients
¼ cup white balsamic vinegar
1 tablespoon Dijon mustard
1 teaspoon sweet paprika
½ teaspoon ground black pepper
¼ teaspoon celery seeds
¼ teaspoon salt
¼ cup olive oil
1½ pounds tiny white potatoes, halved
1 cup blond (white) quinoa
1 medium shallot, minced
2 medium celery stalks, thinly sliced
1 large dill pickle, diced

Directions
1.   Preparing the Ingredients. Whisk the vinegar, mustard, paprika, pepper, celery seeds, and salt in a large serving bowl until smooth; whisk in the olive oil in a thin, steady stream until the dressing is fairly creamy.

Place the potatoes and quinoa in the Multicooker; add enough cold tap water so that the ingredients are submerged by 3 inches (some of the quinoa may float).

2. High pressure for 10 minutes. Lock the lid on the Multicooker and then cook for 10 minutes. To get 10-minutes cook time, press "Pressure" button and use the Time Adjustment button to adjust the cook time to 10 minutes.

3. Pressure Release. Use the quick-release method to bring the pot's pressure back to normal.

4. Finish the dish. Unlock and open the pot. Close the CRISPING LID. Select BROIL, and set the time to 5 minutes. Select START/STOP to begin. Cook until top is browned. Drain the contents of the pot into a colander lined with paper towels or into a fine-mesh sieve in the sink. Do not rinse.

Transfer the potatoes and quinoa to the large bowl with the dressing. Add the shallot, celery, and pickle; toss gently and set aside for a minute or two to warm up the vegetables.

Buttery Carrots With Pancetta

PREP: 5 MINUTES • PRESSURE: 7 MINUTES • BROIL: 5 MINUTES • TOTAL: 17 MINUTES • PRESSURE LEVEL: HIGH • RELEASE: QUICK
SERVES 4 - 6

Ingredients
4 ounces pancetta, diced
1 medium leek, white and pale green parts only, sliced lengthwise, washed, and thinly sliced
¼ cup moderately sweet white wine, such as a dry Riesling
1 pound baby carrots
½ teaspoon ground black pepper
2 tablespoons unsalted butter, cut into small bits

Directions

1. Preparing the Ingredients. Put the pancetta in the Multicooker turned to the "Air crisp" function and use the Time Adjustment button to adjust the cook time to 5 minutes. Add the leek; cook, often stirring, until softened. Pour in the wine and scrape up any browned bits at the bottom of the pot as it comes to a simmer.

Add the carrots and pepper; stir well. Scrape and pour the contents of the Multicooker into a 1-quart, round, high-sided soufflé or baking dish. Dot with the bits of butter. Lay a piece of parchment paper on top of the dish, then a piece of aluminum foil. Seal the foil tightly over the baking dish.

Set the Multicooker rack inside, and pour in 2 cups water. Use aluminum foil to build a sling for the baking dish; lower the baking dish into the cooker.

2. High pressure for 7 minutes. Lock the lid on the Multicooker and then cook for 7 minutes. To get 7-minutes cook time, press "Pressure" button and use the Time Adjustment button to adjust the cook time to 7 minutes.

3. Pressure Release. Use the quick-release method to return the pot's pressure to normal.

4. Finish the dish. Close the CRISPING LID. Select BROIL, and set the time to 5 minutes. Select START/STOP to begin. Cook until top is browned.

Unlock and open the pot. Use the foil sling to lift the baking dish out of the cooker. Uncover, stir well, and serve.

Braised Red Cabbage With Apples

PREP: 5 MINUTES • PRESSURE: 13 MINUTES • BROIL: 23 MINUTES • TOTAL: 18 MINUTES • PRESSURE LEVEL: HIGH • RELEASE: QUICK
SERVES 4

Ingredients
4 thin bacon slices, chopped
1 small red onion, chopped
1 medium tart green apple, such as Granny Smith, peeled, cored, and chopped
1 teaspoon dried thyme
¼ teaspoon ground allspice
¼ teaspoon ground mace
1 tablespoon packed dark brown sugar
1 tablespoon balsamic vinegar
1 medium red cabbage (about 2 pounds), cored and thinly sliced
½ cup chicken broth

Directions
1. Preparing the Ingredients. Fry the bacon in the Multicooker turned to the "air crisp" function, until crisp, about 4 minutes.
Add the onion to the pot; cook, often stirring, until soft, about 4 minutes. Add the apple, thyme, allspice, and mace. Cook about 1 minute, stirring all the while, until fragrant. Stir in the brown sugar and vinegar; keep stirring until bubbling, about 1 minute. Add the cabbage; toss well to mix evenly with the other ingredients. Drizzle the broth over the cabbage mixture.
2. High pressure for 13 minutes. Lock the lid on the Multicooker and then cook for 13 minutes. To get 13-minutes cook time, press "Pressure" button, and use the Time Adjustment button to adjust the cook time to 13 minutes.
3. Pressure Release. Use the quick-release method to return the pot to normal pressure.
Unlock and open the pot.

Close the CRISPING LID. Select BROIL, and set the time to 5 minutes. Select START/STOP to begin. Cook until top is browned. Serve.

Sage-Butter Spaghetti Squash

PREP: 5 MINUTES • PRESSURE: 12 MINUTES • BROIL: 22 MINUTES • TOTAL: 17 MINUTES • PRESSURE LEVEL: HIGH • RELEASE: QUICK
SERVES 6

Ingredients
One 3- to 3½-pound spaghetti squash, halved lengthwise and seeded
6 tablespoons unsalted butter
2 tablespoons packed fresh sage leaves, minced
½ teaspoon salt
½ teaspoon ground black pepper
½ cup finely grated Parmesan cheese (about 1 ounce)

Directions
1. Preparing the Ingredients. Put the squash cut side up in the cooker; add 1 cup water.
2. High pressure for 12 minutes. Lock the lid on the Multicooker and then cook for 12 minutes. To get 12-minutes cook time, press "Pressure" button, and use the Time Adjustment button to adjust the cook time to 12 minutes.
3. Pressure Release. Use the quick-release method to bring the pot's pressure back to normal.
4. Finish the dish. Unlock and open the cooker. Transfer the squash halves to a cutting board; cool for 10 minutes. Discard the liquid in the cooker. Use a fork to scrape the spaghetti-like flesh off the skin and onto the cutting board; discard the skins.
Melt the butter in the electric cooker turned to its browning function. Stir in the sage, salt, and pepper, then add all of the

squash. Stir and toss over the heat until well combined and heated through about 2 minutes. Add the cheese, toss well.

5. Close the CRISPING LID. Select BROIL, and set the time to 5 minutes. Select START/STOP to begin. Cook until top is browned.

Serve.

Parmesan Breaded Zucchini Chips

PREP: 15 MINUTES • COOK TIME: 20 MINUTES • TOTAL: 35 MINUTES
SERVES: 5

Ingredients
For the zucchini chips:
2 medium zucchini
2 eggs
⅓ cup bread crumbs
⅓ cup grated Parmesan cheese
Salt
Pepper
Cooking oil
For the lemon aioli:
½ cup mayonnaise
½ tablespoon olive oil
Juice of ½ lemon
1 teaspoon minced garlic
Salt
Pepper

Directions
1 Preparing the Ingredients. To make the zucchini chips: Slice the zucchini into thin chips (about ⅛ inch thick) using a knife or mandoline.

In a small bowl, beat the eggs. In another small bowl, combine the bread crumbs, Parmesan cheese, and salt and pepper to taste.

Spray the air fryer basket with cooking oil.

Dip the zucchini slices one at a time in the eggs and then the bread crumb mixture. You can also sprinkle the bread crumbs onto the zucchini slices with a spoon.

Place the zucchini chips in the Crisplid-Pot basket, but do not stack.

2   Air Frying. Cook in batches. Spray the chips with cooking oil from a distance (otherwise, the breading may fly off). Cook for 10 minutes.

Remove the cooked zucchini chips from the Crisplid-Pot, then repeat step 5 with the remaining zucchini.

To make the lemon aioli:

While the zucchini is cooking, combine the mayonnaise, olive oil, lemon juice, and garlic in a small bowl, adding salt and pepper to taste. Mix well until fully combined.

Cool the zucchini and serve alongside the aioli.

PER SERVING: CALORIES: 192; FAT: 13G; PROTEIN: 6

Spicy Sweet Potato Fries

PREP: 5 MINUTES • COOK TIME: 37 MINUTES • TOTAL: 45 MINUTES
SERVES: 4

Ingredients
2 tbsp. sweet potato fry seasoning mix
2 tbsp. olive oil
2 sweet potatoes
  Seasoning Mix:

2 tbsp. salt
1 tbsp. cayenne pepper
1 tbsp. dried oregano
1 tbsp. fennel
2 tbsp. coriander

Directions:
1. Preparing the Ingredients. Slice both ends off sweet potatoes and peel. Slice lengthwise in half and again crosswise to make four pieces from each potato.
Slice each potato piece into 2-3 slices, then slice into fries.
Grind together all of seasoning mix ingredients and mix in the salt.
Ensure the Crisplid-Pot is preheated to 350 degrees.
Toss potato pieces in olive oil, sprinkling with seasoning mix and tossing well to coat thoroughly.
2. Air Frying. Add fries to Crisplid-Pot basket. Set temperature to 350°F, and set time to 27 minutes. Select START/STOP to begin.
Take out the basket and turn fries. Turn off Crisplid-Pot and let cook 10-12 minutes till fries are golden.

PER SERVING: CALORIES: 89; FAT: 14G; PROTEIN: 8Gs; SUGAR:3

Air Fried Carrots, Yellow Squash & Zucchini

PREP: 5 MINUTES • COOK TIME: 35 MINUTES • TOTAL: 40 MINUTES
SERVES: 4

Ingredients
1 tbsp. chopped tarragon leaves
½ tsp. white pepper
1 tsp. salt
1 pound yellow squash
1 pound zucchini
6 tsp. olive oil
½ pound carrots

Directions:

1   Preparing the Ingredients. Stem and root the end of squash and zucchini and cut in ¾-inch half-moons. Peel and cut carrots into 1-inch cubes
Combine carrot cubes with 2 teaspoons of olive oil, tossing to combine.
2   Air Frying. Pour into Crisplid-Pot basket, set temperature to 400°F, and set time to 5 minutes.
As carrots cook, drizzle remaining olive oil over squash and zucchini pieces, then season with pepper and salt. Toss well to coat.
Add squash and zucchini when the timer for carrots goes off. Cook 30 minutes, making sure to toss 2-3 times during the cooking process.
Once done, take out veggies and toss with tarragon. Serve up warm!

PER SERVING: CALORIES: 122; FAT: 9G; PROTEIN: 6G; SUGAR:0G

Winter Vegetarian Frittata

PREP: 5 MINUTES • COOK TIME: 30 MINUTES • TOTAL: 35 MINUTES
SERVES: 4

Ingredients
1 leek, peeled and thinly sliced into rings
2 cloves garlic, finely minced
3 medium-sized carrots, finely chopped
2 tablespoons olive oil
6 large-sized eggs
Sea salt and ground black pepper, to taste
1/2 teaspoon dried marjoram, finely minced
1/2 cup yellow cheese of choice

Directions:

1   Preparing the Ingredients. Sauté the leek, garlic, and carrot in hot olive oil until they are tender and fragrant; reserve.
In the meantime, preheat your Crisplid-Pot to 330 degrees F.
In a bowl, whisk the eggs along with the salt, ground black pepper, and marjoram.
Then, grease the inside of your baking dish with a nonstick cooking spray. Pour the whisked eggs into the baking dish. Stir in the sautéed carrot mixture. Top with the cheese shreds.
2   Air Frying. Place the baking dish in the Crisplid-Pot cooking basket. Cook about 30 minutes and serve warm

Air Fried Kale Chips

PREP: 5 MINUTES • COOK TIME: 10 MINUTES • TOTAL: 15 MINUTES
SERVES: 6

Ingredients
¼ tsp. Himalayan salt
3 tbsp. yeast
Avocado oil
1 bunch of kale

Directions:

1. Preparing the Ingredients. Rinse kale and with paper towels, dry well.
Tear kale leaves into large pieces. Remember they will shrink as they cook so good sized pieces are necessary.
Place kale pieces in a bowl and spritz with avocado oil till shiny. Sprinkle with salt and yeast.
With your hands, toss kale leaves well to combine.
2. Air Frying. Pour half of the kale mixture into the Crisplid-Pot, set temperature to 350°F, and set time to 5 minutes. Remove and repeat with another half of kale.

PER SERVING: CALORIES: 55; FAT: 10G; PROTEIN: 1G; SUGAR:0G

Cheesy Cauliflower Fritters

PREP: 10 MINUTES • COOK TIME: 7 MINUTES • TOTAL: 17 MINUTES
SERVES: 8

Ingredients
½ C. chopped parsley
1 C. Italian breadcrumbs
1/3 C. shredded mozzarella cheese
1/3 C. shredded sharp cheddar cheese
1 egg
2 minced garlic cloves
3 chopped scallions
1 head of cauliflower

Directions:
1. Preparing the Ingredients. Cut the cauliflower up into florets. Wash well and pat dry. Place into a food processor and pulse 20-30 seconds till it looks like rice.
Place cauliflower rice in a bowl and mix with pepper, salt, egg, cheeses, breadcrumbs, garlic, and scallions.
With hands, form 15 patties of the mixture. Add more breadcrumbs if needed.
2. Air Frying. With olive oil, spritz patties, and place into your Crisplid-Pot in a single layer. Set temperature to 390°F, and set time to 7 minutes, flipping after 7 minutes.

PER SERVING: CALORIES: 209; FAT: 17G; PROTEIN: 6G; SUGAR:0.5

Roasted Vegetables Salad

PREP: 5 MINUTES • COOK TIME: 85 MINUTES • TOTAL: 90 MINUTES
SERVES: 5

Ingredients

3 eggplants
1 tbsp of olive oil
3 medium zucchini
1 tbsp of olive oil
4 large tomatoes, cut them in eighths
4 cups of one shaped pasta
2 peppers of any color
1 cup of sliced tomatoes cut into small cubes
2 teaspoon of salt substitute
8 tbsp of grated parmesan cheese
½ cup of Italian dressing
Leaves of fresh basil

Directions:
1. Preparing the Ingredients. Wash your eggplant and slice it off then discard the green end. Make sure not to peel.
Slice your eggplant into 1/2 inch of thick rounds. 1/2 inch)
Pour 1tbsp of olive oil on the eggplant round.
2. Air Frying. Put the eggplants in the basket of the Crisplid-Pot and then toss it in the Crisplid-Pot . Cook the eggplants for 40 minutes. Set the heat to 360 ° F
Meanwhile, wash your zucchini and slice it then discard the green end. But do not peel it.
Slice the Zucchini into thick rounds of ½ inch each.
In the basket of the Crisplid-Pot, toss your ingredients
Add 1 tbsp of olive oil.
3. Air Frying. Cook the zucchini for 25 minutes on a heat of 360° F and when the time is off set it aside.
Wash and cut the tomatoes.
4. Air Frying. Arrange your tomatoes in the basket of the Crisplid-Pot. Set the timer to 30 minutes. Set the heat to 350° F

When the time is off, cook your pasta according to the pasta guiding directions, empty it into a colander. Run the cold water on it and wash it and drain the pasta and put it aside.

Meanwhile, wash and chop your peppers and place it in a bow
Wash and thinly slice your cherry tomatoes and add it to the bowl. Add your roasted veggies.

Add the pasta, a pinch of salt, the topping dressing, add the basil and the parm and toss everything together. (It is better to mix with your hands). Set the ingredients together in the refrigerator, and let it chill
Serve your salad and enjoy it!

Zucchini Parmesan Chips

PREP: 10 MINUTES • COOK TIME: 8 MINUTES • TOTAL: 18 MINUTES
SERVES: 10

Ingredients
½ tsp. paprika
½ C. grated parmesan cheese
½ C. Italian breadcrumbs
1 lightly beaten egg
2 thinly sliced zucchinis

Directions:
1   Preparing the Ingredients. Use a very sharp knife or mandolin slicer to slice zucchini as thinly as you can. Pat off extra moisture.
Beat egg with a pinch of pepper and salt and a bit of water.
Combine paprika, cheese, and breadcrumbs in a bowl.
Dip slices of zucchini into the egg mixture and then into breadcrumb mixture. Press gently to coat.
2   Air Frying. With olive oil cooking spray, mist coated zucchini slices. Place into your Crisplid-Pot in a single layer. Set temperature to 350°F, and set time to 8 minutes.

Sprinkle with salt and serve with salsa.

PER SERVING: CALORIES: 211; FAT: 16G; PROTEIN:8G; SUGAR:0G

Vegetable Egg Rolls

PREP: 15 MINUTES • COOK TIME: 10 MINUTES • TOTAL: 25 MINUTES
SERVES: 8

Ingredients

½ cup chopped mushrooms
½ cup grated carrots
½ cup chopped zucchini
2 green onions, chopped
2 tablespoons low-sodium soy sauce
8 egg roll wrappers
1 tablespoon cornstarch
1 egg, beaten

Directions:

1   Preparing the Ingredients. In a medium bowl, combine the mushrooms, carrots, zucchini, green onions, and soy sauce, and stir together. Place the egg roll wrappers on a work surface. Top each with about 3 tablespoons of the vegetable mixture.

In a small bowl, combine the cornstarch and egg and mix well. Brush some of this mixture on the edges of the egg roll wrappers. Roll up the wrappers, enclosing the vegetable filling. Brush some of the egg mixture on the outside of the egg rolls to seal.

2   **Air Frying.** Air-fry for 7 to 10 minutes or until the egg rolls are brown and crunchy.

PER SERVING: CALORIES: 112; FAT: 1G; PROTEIN:4G; FIBER:1G

Buffalo Cauliflower

PREP: 5 MINUTES • COOK TIME: 15 MINUTES • TOTAL: 20 MINUTES
SERVES: 2

Ingredients
Cauliflower:
1 C. panko breadcrumbs
1 tsp. salt
4 C. cauliflower florets
Buffalo Coating:
¼ C. Vegan Buffalo sauce
¼ C. melted vegan butter

Directions:
1   Preparing the Ingredients. Melt butter in microwave and whisk in buffalo sauce.
Dip each cauliflower floret into buffalo mixture, ensuring it gets coated well. Hold over a bowl till floret is done dripping.
Mix breadcrumbs with salt.
2   Air Frying. Dredge dipped florets into breadcrumbs and place into the Crisplid-Pot . Set the temperature to 350°F, and set time to 15 minutes. When slightly browned, they are ready to eat!
Serve with your favorite keto dipping sauce!

PER SERVING: CALORIES: 194; FAT: 17G; PROTEIN:10G; SUGAR:

Jumbo Stuffed Mushrooms

PREP: 10 MINUTES • COOK TIME: 20 MINUTES • TOTAL: 30 MINUTES
SERVES: 4

Ingredients
4 jumbo portobello mushrooms
1 tablespoon olive oil
¼ cup ricotta cheese
5 tablespoons Parmesan cheese, divided
1 cup frozen chopped spinach, thawed and drained
⅓ cup bread crumbs
¼ teaspoon minced fresh rosemary

Directions:

1   Preparing the Ingredients. Wipe the mushrooms with a damp cloth. Remove the stems and discard. Using a spoon, gently scrape out most of the gills.
Rub the mushrooms with the olive oil.
2   Air Frying Put in the Crisplid-Pot basket, hollow side up, and bake for 3 minutes. Carefully remove the mushroom caps, because they will contain liquid. Drain the liquid out of the caps.
In a medium bowl, combine the ricotta, 3 tablespoons of Parmesan cheese, spinach, bread crumbs, and rosemary, and mix well.
Stuff this mixture into the drained mushroom caps. Sprinkle with the remaining 2 tablespoons of Parmesan cheese.
Put the mushroom caps back into the basket and bake for 4 to 6 minutes or until the filling is hot and the mushroom caps are tender.

PER SERVING: CALORIES: 117; FAT: 7G; PROTEIN:7G

Onion Rings

PREP: 10 MINUTES • COOK TIME: 10 MINUTES • TOTAL: 20 MINUTES
SERVES: 4

Ingredients
1 large spanish onion
1/2 cup buttermilk
2 eggs, lightly beaten
3/4 cups unbleached all-purpose flour
3/4 cups panko bread crumbs
1/2 teaspoon baking powder
1/2 teaspoon Cayenne pepper, to taste
Salt

Directions:
1   Preparing the Ingredients. Start by cutting your onion into 1/2 thick rings and separate. Smaller pieces can be discarded or saved for other recipes.
Beat the eggs in a large bowl and mix in the buttermilk, then set it aside.
In another bowl combine flour, pepper, bread crumbs, and baking powder.
Use a large spoon to dip a whole ring in the buttermilk, then pull it through the flour mix on both sides to completely coat the ring.
2   Air Frying. Cook about 8 rings at a time in your Crisplid-Pot for 8-10 minutes at 360 degrees shaking half way through.

PER SERVING: CALORIES: 225; FAT: 3.8G; PROTEIN:19G; FIBER:2.4G

Poultry Recipes

Perfect Chicken Parmesan

PREP: 5 MINUTES • COOK TIME: 25 MINUTES • TOTAL: 30 MINUTES
SERVES: 2

Ingredients
2 large white meat chicken breasts, approximately 5-6 ounces
1 cup of breadcrumbs (Panko brand works well)
2 medium-sized eggs
Pinch of salt and pepper
1 tablespoon of dried oregano
1 cup of marinara sauce (store-bought or homemade will do equally well)
2 slices of provolone cheese
1 tablespoon of parmesan cheese

Directions:
1.   Preparing the Ingredients. Cover the basket of the Crisplid-Pot with a lining of tin foil, leaving the edges uncovered to allow air to circulate through the basket.
Preheat the Crisplid-Pot to 350 degrees.
In a mixing bowl, beat the eggs until fluffy and until the yolks and whites are fully combined, and set aside.
In a separate mixing bowl, combine the breadcrumbs, oregano, salt and pepper, and set aside.

One by one, dip the raw chicken breasts into the bowl with dry ingredients, coating both sides; then submerge into the bowl with wet ingredients, then dip again into the dry ingredients. This double coating will ensure an extra crisp-and-delicious air-fry!

Lay the coated chicken breasts on the foil covering the Crisplid-Pot basket, in a single flat layer.

2.   Air Frying. Set the Crisplid-Pot timer for 10 minutes. After 10 minutes, the Crisplid-Pot will turn off and the chicken should be mid-way cooked and the breaded coating starting to brown.

Using tongs, turn each piece of chicken over to ensure a full all-over fry.

Reset the Crisplid-Pot to 320 degrees for another 10 minutes. While the chicken is cooking, pour half the marinara sauce into a 7-inch heat-safe pan.

After 15 minutes, when the Crisplid-Pot shuts off, remove the fried chicken breasts using tongs and set in the marinara-covered pan. Drizzle the rest of the marinara sauce over the fried chicken, then place the slices of provolone cheese atop both of them and sprinkle the parmesan cheese over the entire pan.

Reset the Crisplid-Pot to 350 degrees for 5 minutes.

After 5 minutes, when the Crisplid-Pot shuts off, remove the dish from the Crisplid-Pot using tongs or oven mitts. The chicken will be perfectly crisped and the cheese melted and lightly toasted. Serve while hot!

Enchilada-Braised Chicken Breasts

PREP: 5 MINUTES • PRESSURE: 15 MINUTES • AIR CRISP: 9 MINUTES • TOTAL: 29 MINUTES • PRESSURE LEVEL: HIGH • RELEASE: QUICK
SERVES 4

Ingredients
1 teaspoon packed dark brown sugar
1 teaspoon ground cumin
1 teaspoon smoked paprika
½ teaspoon salt
½ teaspoon ground black pepper
½ teaspoon onion powder
¼ teaspoon garlic powder
Four 6- to 8-ounce boneless skinless chicken breasts
2 tablespoons olive oil
One 8-ounce can tomato sauce (1 cup)
½ cup light-colored beer, preferably a Pilsner or an IPA
2 tablespoons chili powder
2 tablespoons fresh lime juice

Directions
1. Preparing the Ingredients. Mix the brown sugar, cumin, smoked paprika, salt, pepper, onion powder, and garlic powder in a medium bowl. Massage the spice rub onto the chicken breasts.
Heat the oil in the Multicooker using the "Sauté" function. Set the breasts in the cooker and brown well, turning once, about 6 minutes.
Mix the tomato sauce, beer, chili powder, and lime juice in the bowl the spices were in; pour the sauce over the breasts.
2. High pressure for 15 minutes. Close the lid and Cook for 15 minutes. To get 15-minutes cook time, press the "Pressure" Button and adjust the time.
3. Pressure Release. Use the quick-release method to bring the pot's pressure back to normal.

4. Close CRISPING LID. Select AIR CRISP, set temperature to 390°F, and set time to 9 minutes. Check after 6 minutes, cooking for an additional 3 minutes if dish needs more browning. Serve the chicken with the sauce ladled on top.

Honey-Chipotle Chicken Wings

PREP: 5 MINUTES • PRESSURE: 10 MINUTES • AIR CRISP: 10 MINUTES • TOTAL: 25 MINUTES • PRESSURE LEVEL: HIGH • RELEASE: QUICK
SERVES 2

Ingredients
1 cup water, for steaming
3 tablespoons Mexican hot sauce (such as Valentina brand)
2 tablespoons honey
1 teaspoon minced canned chipotle in adobo sauce

Directions
1. Preparing the Ingredients. If using whole wings, cut off the tips and discard. Cut the wings at the joint into two pieces each, the "drumette" and the "flat."
Add the water and insert the steamer basket or trivet. Place the wings on the steamer insert.
2. High pressure for 10 minutes. Close the lid and the pressure valve and then cook for 10 minutes. To get 10-minutes cook time, press "Pressure" button and the time selector.
3. Pressure Release. Use the quick-release method.
4. Finish the dish. While the wings are cooking, make the sauce. In a large bowl, whisk together the hot sauce, honey, and minced chipotle.
5. Close crisping lid. Select AIR CRISP, set temperature to 390°F, and set time to 10 minutes. Select START/STOP to begin. Serve!

PER SERVING: CALORIES: 434; FAT: 27G; SODIUM: 1,152MG; CARBOHYDRATES: 19G; FIBER: 1G; PROTEIN: 31G

Lemon and Olive Ligurian Chicken

PREP: 10 MINUTES • PRESSURE: 15 MINUTES • AIR CRISP: 10 MINUTES • TOTAL: 35 MINUTES • PRESSURE LEVEL: HIGH • RELEASE: NORMAL
SERVES 6-8

Ingredients
2 garlic cloves, chopped
3 sprigs of Fresh Rosemary (two for chopping, one for garnish)
2 sprigs of Fresh Sage
½ bunch of Parsley Leaves and stems
3 lemons, juiced (about a ¾ cup or 180ml)
4 tablespoons extra virgin olive oil
1 teaspoon sea salt
¼ teaspoon pepper
1 whole chicken, cut into parts or package of bone-in chicken pieces, skin removed (or not) ½ cup (125ml) dry white wine
3.5oz (100g) Black Gourmet Salt-Cured Olives (Taggiesche, French, or Kalamata)
1 fresh lemon, for garnish (optional)

Directions
1. Preparing the Ingredients. Prepare the marinade by finely chopping together the garlic, rosemary, sage, and parsley.

Place them in a container and add the lemon juice, olive oil, salt, and pepper. Mix well and set aside.

Remove the skin from the chicken (save it for a chicken stock).

In the preheated Multicooker, with the lid off, add a swirl of olive oil and brown the chicken pieces on all sides for about 5 minutes.

De-glaze cooker with the white wine until it has almost all evaporated (about 3 minutes).

Add the chicken pieces back in - this time being careful with the order. Put all dark-meat (wings, legs, thighs) first, and then the chicken breasts on top so that they do not touch the bottom of the Multicooker.

Pour the remaining marinade on top. Don't worry if this does not seem like enough liquid, the chicken will also release its juices into the cooker, too.

2. High pressure for 10 minutes. Lock the lid on the Multicooker and then cook for 10 minutes. To get 10-minutes cook time, press "Pressure" button and adjust the time.

3. Pressure Release. When time is up, open the cooker by releasing the pressure using the Quick-Release Method.

5. Finish the dish. Close crisping lid. Select AIR CRISP, set temperature to 390°F, and set time to 10 minutes. Check after 5 minutes, cooking for an additional 5 minutes if dish needs more browning.

Take the chicken pieces out of the cooker and place on a serving platter tightly covered with foil.

Reduce the cooking liquid in the Multicooker, if necessary, with the lid off to ¼ of its amount, or until it becomes thick and syrupy.

Put all of the chicken pieces back into the Multicooker to warm up. Mix and spoon the thick glaze onto the chicken pieces and simmer it in the glaze for a few minutes before serving.

Sprinkle with fresh rosemary, olives and lemon slices. When serving, caution your guests that the olives still have their pits!

Per Serving Calories: 204.8; Fat: 12.2g; Carbohydrates: 3.1g; Sugar: 0.7g; Fiber: 0.3g; Protein: 17.8g; Sodium: 449.5mg; Cholesterol: 61.6mg

Honey Soy Chicken Wings

PREP: 10 MINUTES • PRESSURE: 20 MINUTES • AIR CRISP: 10 MINUTES • TOTAL: 40 MINUTES • PRESSURE LEVEL: HIGH • RELEASE: NATURAL
SERVES 2-4

Ingredients
1 ½ pound chicken wings
4 cloves garlic, roughly minced
½ large shallot or 1 small shallot, roughly minced
1 – 2 star anise
1 tablespoon ginger, sliced
1 tablespoon honey
½ cup warm water
1 tablespoon peanut oil
1 ½ tablespoon cornstarch
Chicken Wing Marinade
2 tablespoons light soy sauce
1 tablespoon dark soy sauce
1 tablespoon Shaoxing wine
1 teaspoon sugar
¼ teaspoon salt

Directions
1.   Preparing the Ingredients. Marinate the chicken wings with the Chicken Wing Marinade for 20 minutes.

Heat the Multicooker using the "Sauté" function.

Add 1 tablespoon of peanut oil into the pot. Add the marinated chicken wings into the pot. Then, brown the chicken wings for roughly 30 seconds on each side. Flip a few times as you brown them as the soy sauce and sugar can be burnt easily. Remove and set aside.

Add the minced shallot, star anise and sliced ginger, then stir for roughly a minute. Add the minced garlic and stir until fragrant (roughly 30 seconds).

Mix 1 tablespoon of honey with ½ cup of warm water, then add it into the pot and deglaze the bottom of the pot with a wooden spoon.

Place all the chicken wings with all the meat juice and the leftover chicken wing marinade into the pot.

2. High pressure for 5 minutes. Lock the lid on the Multicooker and then cook for 5 minutes. To get 5-minutes cook time, press "Pressure" button and use the Time Adjustment button to adjust the cook time to 5 minutes.

3. Pressure Release. Let the pressure to come down naturally for at least 10 minutes, then quick release any pressure left in the pot.

4. Finish the dish. Close crisping lid. Select AIR CRISP, set temperature to 390°F, and set time to 10 minutes. Check after 10 minutes, cooking for an additional 5 minutes if dish needs more browning.

Open the lid carefully and taste one of the honey soy chicken wings and the honey soy sauce. Season with more salt or honey if desired.

Remove all the chicken wings from the pot and set aside. Turn the Multicooker to its sauté function. Mix 1 ½ tablespoon of cornstarch with 1 tablespoon of cold running tap water. Keep mixing and add it into the honey soy sauce one third at a time until desired thickness.

Turn off the heat and add the chicken wings back into the pot. Coat well with the honey soy sauce and serve immediately!

Thai Green Chicken Curry

PREP: 15 MINUTES • PRESSURE: 10 MINUTES • AIR CRISP: 10 MINUTES • TOTAL: 25 MINUTES • PRESSURE LEVEL: HIGH • RELEASE: QUICK
SERVES 6-8

Ingredients
1 tablespoon vegetable oil
1 medium onion, peeled, and sliced thin
3 cloves garlic, crushed
1/2 inch piece of ginger, peeled and crushed
Cream from the top of a (13.5 ounce) can coconut milk
4 tablespoons green curry paste (a whole 4 oz. can)
3 pounds boneless skinless chicken thighs, cut into 1/2 inch by 2 inch lengths
1 teaspoon Diamond Crystal kosher salt or 3/4 teaspoon fine sea salt
The rest of the (13.5 ounce) can coconut milk
1 cup chicken stock or water
1 tablespoon fish sauce (plus more to taste)
1 tablespoon soy sauce (plus more to taste)
1 tablespoon brown sugar (plus more to taste)
Juice from 1 lime
12 ounces green beans, trimmed and cut into 2 inch pieces
Minced cilantro
Minced basil (preferably Thai basil)
Lime wedges
Jasmine rice

Directions

1. Preparing the Ingredients. Heat the vegetable oil in the Multicooker until shimmering, use Sauté mode. Stir in the onion, garlic, and ginger, and Sauté until the onion starts to soften, about 3 minutes.

Fry the curry paste: Scoop the cream from the top of the can of coconut milk and add it to the pot, then stir in the curry paste. Cook, often stirring, until the curry paste darkens, about 5 minutes.

Sprinkle the chicken with the kosher salt. Add the chicken to the pot, and stir to coat with curry paste. Stir in the rest of the can of coconut milk, chicken stock, fish sauce, soy sauce, and brown sugar.

2. High pressure for 10 minutes. Lock the lid on the Multicooker and then cook for 10 minutes. To get 10-minutes cook time, press "Pressure" button and use the Time Adjustment button to adjust the cook time to 10 minutes.

3. Pressure Release. Use the quick-release method to bring the pot's pressure back to normal.

4. Finish the dish. Close crisping lid. Select AIR CRISP, set temperature to 390°F, and set time to 15 minutes. Check after 10 minutes, cooking for an additional 5 minutes if dish needs more browning.

Finish the curry: Remove the lid from the Multicooker, then set Sauté mode. Stir in the lime juice and the green beans, and simmer the curry until the green beans are crisp-tender, about 4 minutes. Taste the curry for seasoning, adding more soy sauce (to add salt) or brown sugar (to add sweet) as needed. Ladle the curry into bowls, sprinkle with minced cilantro and basil, and serve with Jasmine rice.

Enjoy

Chicken-Fried Steak Supreme

PREP: 10 MINUTES • COOK TIME: 30 MINUTES • TOTAL: 40 MINUTES
SERVES: 8

Ingredients
½ pound beef-bottom round, sliced into strips
1 cup of breadcrumbs (Panko brand works well)
2 medium-sized eggs
Pinch of salt and pepper
½ tablespoon of ground thyme

Directions:

1. Preparing the Ingredients. Cover the basket of the Crisplid-Pot with a lining of tin foil, leaving the edges uncovered to allow air to circulate through the basket. Preheat the Crisplid-Pot to 350 degrees. In a mixing bowl, beat the eggs until fluffy and until the yolks and whites are fully combined, and set aside. In a separate mixing bowl, combine the breadcrumbs, thyme, salt and pepper, and set aside. One by one, dip each piece of raw steak into the bowl with dry ingredients, coating all sides; then submerge into the bowl with wet ingredients, then dip again into the dry ingredients. This double coating will ensure an extra crisp air fry. Lay the coated steak pieces on the foil covering the air-fryer basket, in a single flat layer.

2. Air Frying. Set the Crisplid-Pot timer for 15 minutes. After 15 minutes, the Crisplid-Pot will turn off and the steak should be mid-way cooked and the breaded coating starting to brown. Using tongs, turn each piece of steak over to ensure a full all-over fry. Reset the Crisplid-Pot to 320 degrees for 15 minutes. After 15 minutes, when the Crisplid-Pot shuts off, remove the fried steak strips using tongs and set on a serving plate. Eat as soon as cool enough to handle and enjoy!

Lemon-Pepper Chicken Wings

PREP: 10 MINUTES • COOK TIME: 20 MINUTES • TOTAL: 30 MINUTES
SERVES: 4

Ingredients
8 whole chicken wings
Juice of ½ lemon
½ teaspoon garlic powder
1 teaspoon onion powder
Salt
Pepper
¼ cup low-fat buttermilk
½ cup all-purpose flour
Cooking oil

Directions:
1. Preparing the Ingredients. Place the wings in a sealable plastic bag. Drizzle the wings with the lemon juice. Season the wings with the garlic powder, onion powder, and salt and pepper to taste.
Seal the bag. Shake thoroughly to combine the seasonings and coat the wings.
Pour the buttermilk and the flour into separate bowls large enough to dip the wings.
Spray the Crisplid-Pot basket with cooking oil.
One at a time, dip the wings in the buttermilk and then the flour.
2. Air Frying. Place the wings in the Crisplid-Pot basket. It is okay to stack them on top of each other. Spray the wings with cooking oil, being sure to spray the bottom layer. Cook for 5 minutes.
Remove the basket and shake it to ensure all of the pieces will cook fully.

Return the basket to the Crisplid-Pot and continue to cook the chicken. Repeat shaking every 5 minutes until a total of 20 minutes has passed.
Cool before serving.

PER SERVING: CALORIES: 347; FAT: 12G; PROTEIN:46G; FIBER:1G

Easy Turkey Breast

PREP: 10 MINUTES • PRESSURE: 60 MINUTES • TOTAL: 70 MINUTES • PRESSURE LEVEL: HIGH • RELEASE: NATURAL
SERVES 4

Ingredients
1 frozen turkey breast with frozen gravy packet
1 whole onion

Directions
1. Preparing the Ingredients. Place frozen turkey breast, rozen gravy packet and whole onion in the Multicooker.
2. High pressure for 30 minutes. Lock the lid on the Multicooker and then cook for 30 minutes. To get 30-minutes cook time, press "Pressure" button and use the Time Adjustment button to adjust the cook time to 30 minutes.
3. Pressure Release. Use natural-release method.
Remove lid, turn turkey breast over
4. High pressure for 30 minutes. Replace lid on the Multicooker and then cook for 30 minutes. To get 30-minutes cook time, press "Pressure" button
and use the Time Adjustment button to adjust the cook time to 30 minutes.
5. Pressure Release. Use natural-release method, again.
6. Finish the dish. Close crisping lid. Select AIR CRISP, set temperature to 360°F, and set time to 10 minutes. Check after 5 minutes, cooking for an additional 5 minutes if dish needs more browning.
Remove mesh. Remove turkey and slice. Places slices and turkey gravy into serving dish.
Enjoy

Turkey Breast

PREP: 20 MINUTES • PRESSURE: 45 MINUTES • AIR CRISP: 15 MINUTES • TOTAL: 80 MINUTES • PRESSURE LEVEL: HIGH • RELEASE: NATURAL & QUICK
SERVES 4

Ingredients
6.5 lb. bone-in, skin-on turkey breast
Salt and pepper, to taste
1 (14 oz.) can turkey or chicken broth
1 large onion, quartered
1 stock celery, cut in large pieces
1 sprig thyme
3 tablespoons cornstarch
3 tablespoons cold water

Directions
1. Preparing the Ingredients. Season turkey breast liberally with salt and pepper.
Put trivet in the bottom. Add chicken broth, onion, celery and thyme. Add the turkey to the cooking pot breast side up.
2. High pressure for 45 minutes. Lock the lid on the Multicooker and then cook for 45 minutes. To get 45-minutes cook time, press "Pressure" button and use the adjust button to adjust the cook time to 45 minutes.
3. Pressure Release. Use a natural pressure release for 10 minutes, then do a quick pressure release.
Check if the turkey is done. If it isn't, lock the lid in place and cook it for a few more minutes.

4. Finish the dish. Close crisping lid. Select AIR CRISP, set temperature to 360°F, and set time to 10 minutes. Check after 5 minutes, cooking for an additional 5 minutes if dish needs more browning. Carefully remove turkey and place on large plate. Cover with foil.

Strain and skim the fat off the broth. Whisk together cornstarch and cold water; add to broth in cooking pot. Select Sauté and stir until broth thickens.

Add salt and pepper to taste.

Slice the turkey and serve immediately.

Enjoy!

Paleo Turkey and Gluten-Free Gravy

PREP: 10 MINUTES • PRESSURE: 35 MINUTES • TOTAL: 55 MINUTES • PRESSURE LEVEL: HIGH • RELEASE: QUICK SERVES 6

Ingredients
1 4-5 pound bone-in, skin-on turkey breast
Salt
Black pepper (omit for AIP)
2 tablespoons ghee or butter (use coconut oil for AIP)
1 medium onion, cut into medium dice
1 large carrot, cut into medium dice
1 celery rib, cut into medium dice
1 garlic clove, peeled and smashed
2 teaspoons dried sage
¼ cup dry white wine
1½ cups bone broth (preferably from chicken or turkey bones)
1 bay leaf
1 tablespoon tapioca starch (optional)

Directions
1. Preparing the Ingredients. Set the "Sauté" function.

Pat turkey breast dry and generously season with salt and pepper. Melt cooking fat in the Multicooker.

Brown turkey breast, skin side down, about 5 minutes, and transfer to a plate, leaving fat in the pot.

Add onion, carrot, and celery to pot and cook until softened, about 5 minutes. Stir in garlic and sage and cook until fragrant, about 30 seconds.

Pour in wine and cook until slightly reduced about 3 minutes. Stir in broth and bay leaf. Using a wooden spoon, scrape up all browned bits stuck on the bottom of pot.

Place turkey skin side up in the pot with any accumulated juices.

2. High pressure for 35 minutes. Lock the lid on the Multicooker and then cook for 35 minutes. To get 35-minutes cook time, press "Pressure" button, and use the Time Adjustment button to adjust the cook time to 35

3. Pressure Release. Use quick-release method and carefully remove lid.

4. Finish the dish. Close crisping lid. Select AIR CRISP, set temperature to 375°F, and set time to 10 minutes. Check after 5 minutes, cooking for an additional 5 minutes if dish needs more browning.

Transfer turkey breast to carving board or plate and tent loosely with foil, allowing it to rest while you prepare the gravy.

Use an immersion blender or carefully transfer cooking liquid and vegetables to blender and puree until smooth. Return to heat and cook until thickened and reduced to about 2 cups. Adjust seasoning to taste.

Slice turkey breast and serve with hot gravy. Enjoy

Minty Chicken-Fried Pork Chops

PREP: 10 MINUTES • COOK TIME: 30 MINUTES • TOTAL: 40 MINUTES
SERVES: 6

Ingredients
4 medium-sized pork chops, approximately 3.5 ounces each
1 cup of breadcrumbs (Panko brand works well)
2 medium-sized eggs
Pinch of salt and pepper
½ tablespoon of mint, either dried and ground; or fresh, rinsed and finely chopped

Directions:
1.	Preparing the Ingredients. Cover the basket of the Crisplid-Pot with a lining of tin foil, leaving the edges uncovered to allow air to circulate through the basket. Preheat the Crisplid-Pot to 350 degrees.
In a mixing bowl, beat the eggs until fluffy and until the yolks and whites are fully combined, and set aside.
In a separate mixing bowl, combine the breadcrumbs, mint, salt, and pepper, and set aside. One by one, dip each raw pork chop into the bowl with dry ingredients, coating all sides; then submerge into the bowl with wet ingredients, then dip again into the dry ingredients. This double coating will ensure an extra crisp air-fry. Lay the coated pork chops on the foil covering the Crisplid-Pot basket, in a single flat layer.
2.	Air Frying. Set the Crisplid-Pot timer for 15 minutes. After 15 minutes, the Crisplid-Pot will turn off, and the pork should be mid-way cooked and the breaded coating starting to brown. Using tongs, turn each piece of steak over to ensure a full all-over fry. Reset the Crisplid-Pot to 320 degrees for 15 minutes.

After 15 minutes, when the Crisplid-Pot shuts off, remove the fried pork chops using tongs and set on a serving plate. Eat as soon as cool enough to handle – and enjoy

Crispy Southern Fried Chicken

PREP: 10 MINUTES • COOK TIME: 25 MINUTES • TOTAL: 35 MINUTES
SERVES: 4

Ingredients
1 tsp. cayenne pepper
2 tbsp. mustard powder
2 tbsp. oregano
2 tbsp. thyme
3 tbsp. coconut milk
1 beaten egg
¼ C. cauliflower
¼ C. gluten-free oats
8 chicken drumsticks

Directions:
1. Preparing the Ingredients. Ensure the Crisplid-Pot is preheated to 350 degrees.
Lay out chicken and season with pepper and salt on all sides.
Add all other ingredients to a blender, blending till a smooth-like breadcrumb mixture is created. Place in a bowl and add a beaten egg to another bowl.
Dip chicken into breadcrumbs, then into the egg, and breadcrumbs once more.
2. Air Frying. Place coated drumsticks into the Crisplid-Pot. Set temperature to 350°F, and set time to 20 minutes and cook

20 minutes. Bump up the temperature to 390 degrees and cook another 5 minutes till crispy.

PER SERVING: CALORIES: 504; FAT: 18G; PROTEIN:35G; SUGAR:5G

Tex-Mex Turkey Burgers

PREP: 10 MINUTES • COOK TIME: 15 MINUTES • TOTAL: 25 MINUTES
SERVES: 4

Ingredients
⅓ cup finely crushed corn tortilla chips
1 egg, beaten
¼ cup salsa
⅓ cup shredded pepper Jack cheese
Pinch salt
Freshly ground black pepper
1 pound ground turkey
1 tablespoon olive oil
1 teaspoon paprika

Directions:
1.   Preparing the Ingredients. In a medium bowl, combine the tortilla chips, egg, salsa, cheese, salt, and pepper, and mix well.
Add the turkey and mix gently but thoroughly with clean hands. Form the meat mixture into patties about ½ inch thick. Make an indentation in the center of each patty with your thumb, so the burgers don't puff up while cooking.

Brush the patties on both sides with the olive oil and sprinkle with paprika.

2. Air Frying. Put in the Crisplid-Pot basket. Grill for 14 to 16 minutes or until the meat registers at least 165°F.

PER SERVING: CALORIES: 354; FAT: 21G; PROTEIN:36G; FIBER:2G

Air Fryer Turkey Breast

PREP: 5 MINUTES • COOK TIME: 60 MINUTES • TOTAL: 65 MINUTES
SERVES: 6

Ingredients
Pepper and salt
1 oven-ready turkey breast
Turkey seasonings of choice

Directions:
1   Preparing the Ingredients. Preheat the Crisplid-Pot to 350 degrees.
Season turkey with pepper, salt, and other desired seasonings. Place turkey in the Crisplid-Pot basket.
2   Air Frying. Set temperature to 350°F, and set time to 60 minutes. Cook 60 minutes. The meat should be at 165 degrees when done.
Allow to rest 10-15 minutes before slicing. Enjoy

PER SERVING: CALORIES: 212; FAT: 12G; PROTEIN:24G; SUGAR:0G

Chicken Nuggets

PREP: 10 MINUTES • COOK TIME: 20 MINUTES • TOTAL: 30 MINUTES
SERVES: 4

Ingredients
1 pound boneless, skinless chicken breasts
Chicken seasoning or rub
Salt
Pepper
2 eggs
6 tablespoons bread crumbs
2 tablespoons panko bread crumbs
Cooking oil

Directions:
1. Preparing the Ingredients. Cut the chicken breasts into 1-inch pieces.
In a large bowl, combine the chicken pieces with chicken seasoning, salt, and pepper to taste.
In a small bowl, beat the eggs. In another bowl, combine the bread crumbs and panko.
Dip the chicken pieces in the eggs and then the bread crumbs.
Place the nuggets in the Crisplid-Pot. Do not overcrowd the basket. Cook in batches. Spray the nuggets with cooking oil.
2. Air Frying. Cook for 4 minutes. Open the Crisplid-Pot and shake the basket. Cook for an additional 4 minutes. Remove the cooked nuggets from the Crisplid-Pot then repeat steps 5 and 6 for the remaining chicken nuggets. Cool before serving.

PER SERVING: CALORIES: 206; FAT: 5G; PROTEIN:31G; FIBER:1G

Cheesy Chicken Fritters

PREP: 5 MINUTES • COOK TIME: 20 MINUTES • TOTAL: 25 MINUTES
SERVES: 17 FRITTERS

Ingredients
    Chicken Fritters:
    ½ tsp. salt
    1/8 tsp. pepper
    1 ½ tbsp. fresh dill
    1 1/3 C. shredded mozzarella cheese
    1/3 C. coconut flour
    1/3 C. vegan mayo
    2 eggs
    1 ½ pounds chicken breasts
    Garlic Dip:
    1/8 tsp. pepper
    ¼ tsp. salt
    ½ tbsp. lemon juice
    1 pressed garlic cloves
    1/3 C. vegan mayo

Directions:

1   Preparing the Ingredients. Slice chicken breasts into 1/3" pieces and place in a bowl. Add all remaining fritter ingredients to the bowl and stir well. Cover and chill 2 hours or overnight. Ensure your Crisplid-Pot is preheated to 350 degrees. Spray basket with a bit of olive oil.

2   Air Frying. Add marinated chicken to the Crisplid-Pot. Set temperature to 350°F, and set time to 20 minutes and cook 20 minutes, making sure to turn halfway through cooking process.

To make the dipping sauce, combine all the dip ingredients until smooth.

PER SERVING: CALORIES: 467; FAT: 27G; PROTEIN:21G; SUGAR:3G

Air Fryer Chicken Parmesan

PREP: 5 MINUTES • COOK TIME: 9 MINUTES • TOTAL: 20 MINUTES
SERVES: 4

Ingredients
- ½ C. keto marinara
- 6 tbsp. mozzarella cheese
- 1 tbsp. melted ghee
- 2 tbsp. grated parmesan cheese
- 6 tbsp. gluten-free seasoned breadcrumbs
- 1   8-ounce chicken breasts

Directions:
1   Preparing the Ingredients. Ensure Crisplid-Pot is preheated to 360 degrees. Spray the basket with olive oil.
Mix parmesan cheese and breadcrumbs together. Melt ghee. Brush melted ghee onto the chicken and dip into breadcrumb mixture.
Place coated chicken in the Crisplid-Pot and top with olive oil.
2   Air Frying. Set temperature to 360°F, and set time to 6 minutes. Cook 2 breasts for 6 minutes and top each breast with a tablespoon of sauce and 1½ tablespoons of mozzarella cheese. Cook another 3 minutes to melt cheese.

Keep cooked pieces warm as you repeat the process with remaining breasts.

PER SERVING: CALORIES: 251; FAT: 10G; PROTEIN:31G; SUGAR:0G

Ricotta and Parsley Stuffed Turkey Breasts

PREP: 5 MINUTES • COOK TIME: 25 MINUTES • TOTAL: 30 MINUTES
SERVES: 4

Ingredients
- 1 turkey breast, quartered
- 1 cup Ricotta cheese
- 1/4 cup fresh Italian parsley, chopped
- 1 teaspoon garlic powder
- 1/2 teaspoon cumin powder
- 1 egg, beaten
- 1 teaspoon paprika
- Salt and ground black pepper, to taste
- Crushed tortilla chips
- 1 ½ tablespoons extra-virgin olive oil

Directions:

1. Preparing the Ingredients. Firstly, flatten out each piece of turkey breast with a rolling pin. Prepare three mixing bowls.
In a shallow bowl, combine Ricotta cheese with the parsley, garlic powder, and cumin powder.
Place the Ricotta/parsley mixture in the middle of each piece. Repeat with the remaining pieces of the turkey breast and roll them up.
In another shallow bowl, whisk the egg together with paprika. In the third shallow bowl, combine the salt, pepper, and crushed tortilla chips.
Dip each roll in the whisked egg, then, roll them over the tortilla chips mixture.
Transfer prepared rolls to the Crisplid-Pot basket. Drizzle olive oil over all.
2. Air Frying. Cook at 350 degrees F for 25 minutes, working in batches. Serve warm, garnished with some extra parsley, if

desired.

Pork Recipes

Pork Shoulder Chops With Soy Sauce, Maple Syrup, And Carrots
PREP: 5 MINUTES • PRESSURE: 40 MINUTES • BROIL: 7 MINUTES • TOTAL: 52 MINUTES • PRESSURE LEVEL: HIGH • RELEASE: NATURAL
SERVES 6

Ingredients
1 tablespoon bacon fat
3 pounds bone-in pork shoulder chops, each ½ to ¾ inch thick
6 medium carrots
3 medium garlic cloves
⅓ cup soy sauce
⅓ cup maple syrup
⅓ cup chicken broth
½ teaspoon ground black pepper

Directions
1. Preparing the Ingredients. Melt the bacon fat in a Multicooker, turned to the browning function. Add about half the chops and brown well, turning once, about 5 minutes. Transfer these to a large bowl and brown the remaining chops. Stir the carrots and garlic into the pot; cook for 1 minute, constantly stirring. Pour in the soy sauce, maple syrup, and broth, stirring to dissolve the maple syrup and to get up any browned bits on the bottom of the pot. Stir in the pepper.

Return the shoulder chops and their juices to the pot. Stir to coat them in the sauce.

2. High pressure for 40 minutes. Lock the lid on the Multicooker and then cook for 40 minutes. To get 40-minutes cook time, press "Pressure" button and use the Time Adjustment button to adjust the cook time to 40 minutes.

3. Pressure Release. Let the pressure to come down naturally for at least 14 to 16 minutes, then quick release any pressure left in the pot.

4. Finish the dish. Close CRISPING LID and select Broil, set time to 7 minutes.

Transfer the chops, carrots, and garlic cloves to a large serving bowl. Skim the fat off the sauce and ladle it over the servings.

Pulled Pork

PREP: 5 MINUTES • PRESSURE: 80 MINUTES • BROIL: 7 MINUTES • TOTAL: 92 MINUTES • PRESSURE LEVEL: HIGH • RELEASE: NATURAL
SERVES 8

Ingredients
2 tablespoons smoked paprika
2 tablespoons packed dark brown sugar
1 tablespoon ground cumin
2 teaspoons ground black pepper
½ tablespoon dry mustard
1 teaspoon ground coriander
1 teaspoon dried thyme
1 teaspoon onion powder
1 teaspoon salt
½ teaspoon garlic powder
½ teaspoon ground cloves

½ teaspoon ground cinnamon

One 4- to 4½-pound bone-in skinless pork shoulder, preferably pork butt

Up to 1½ cups light-colored beer, preferably a pale ale or amber lager

Directions

1. Preparing the Ingredients. Mix the smoked paprika, brown sugar, cumin, pepper, mustard, coriander, thyme, onion powder, salt, garlic powder, cloves, and cinnamon in a small bowl. Massage the mixture all over the pork.

Set the pork in the Multicooker. Pour 1cup beer into the electric cooker without knocking the spices off the meat.

2. High pressure for 80 minutes. Lock the lid on the Multicooker and then cook for 80 minutes. To get 80-minutes cook time, press "Pressure" button and use the Time Adjustment button to adjust the cook time to 80 minutes.

3. Pressure Release. Let its pressure fall to normal naturally, 25 to 35 minutes.

4. Finish the dish. Close CRISPING LID and select Broil, set time to 7 minutes.

5. Transfer the meat to a large cutting board. Let stand for 5 minutes. Use a spoon to skim as much fat off the sauce in the pot as possible.

Set the "Saute" function. Bring the sauce to a simmer, stirring occasionally; continue boiling the sauce, often stirring, until reduced by half, 7 to 10 minutes.

Use two forks to shred the meat off the bones; discard the bones and any attached cartilage. Pull any large chunks of meat apart with the forks and stir the meat back into the simmering sauce to reheat.

Serve and Enjoy

Crispy Pork Carnitas

PREP: 15 MINUTES • PRESSURE: 50 MINUTES • BROIL: 7 MINUTES • TOTAL: 72 MINUTES • PRESSURE LEVEL: HIGH • RELEASE: NATURAL
SERVES 11

Ingredients
2 1/2 pounds trimmed, boneless pork shoulder blade roast
2 teaspoons kosher salt
black pepper, to taste
6 cloves garlic, cut into sliver
1 1/2 teaspoons cumin
1/2 teaspoon sazon
1/4 teaspoon dry oregano
3/4 cup reduced-sodium chicken broth
2-3 chipotle peppers in adobo sauce (to taste)
2 bay leaves
1/4 teaspoon dry adobo seasoning
1/2 teaspoon garlic powder

Directions
1. Preparing the Ingredients. Season pork with salt and pepper. Bring the cooker to high pressure by pressing the Sauté button, and brown pork on all sides on high heat for about 5 minutes. Remove from heat and allow to cool.
Using a sharp knife, insert blade into pork about 1-inch deep, and insert the garlic slivers, you'll want to do this all over. Season pork with cumin, sazon, oregano, adobo and garlic powder all over.
Pour chicken broth, add chipotle peppers and stir, add bay leaves and place pork in the Multicooker.
2. High pressure for 50 minutes. Lock the lid on the Multicooker and then cook for 50 minutes. To get 50-minutes

cook time, press "Pressure" button and use the Time Adjustment button to adjust the cook time to 50 minutes.
3. Pressure Release. Use natural-release method. Close crisping lid and select Broil, set time to 7 minutes.
Serve and Enjoy!

Per Serving Calories: 160; Fat: 7g; Sat Fat: 3g; Carb: 1g; Fiber: 0g; Protein: 20g; Sugar: 0g; Sodium: 397 mg; Cholesterol: 69mg

Easy Pork Chops

PREP: 15 MINUTES • PRESSURE: 5 MINUTES • BROIL: 7 MINUTES • TOTAL: 27 MINUTES • PRESSURE LEVEL: LOW • RELEASE: NATURAL
SERVES 6

Ingredients
3-4 Pork Chops – ½ to ¾ inch thick
One egg – beaten
Flour
Salt and Pepper
Bread Crumbs
Onions – chopped – as much as you like – ½ cup maybe
2 – 4 Garlic cloves – squashed and chopped
Butter- 1 tbsp.
Oil 1-2 tbsp. or orange/ginger coconut oil

Directions
1. Preparing the Ingredients. Turn on the Multicooker to the Sauté setting, then wait for it to boil. Heat the oil and butter to very hot.
Make sure your pork chops are at room temperature. Dredge them in flour, dip into beaten egg, dredge them in bread

crumbs. Brown them lots on both sides in the hot Multicooker. When well browned on both sides, remove and put on the plate.

Throw in the onions, swish them around for a minute until softer looking, then throw in the garlic and swish around.

Leave the onions, garlic, and drippings in the pot. Add about two to three tablespoons of water. Put steamer in the pot, place browned pork chops on steamer above the water and drippings.

2. High pressure for 5 minutes. Lock the lid on the Multicooker and then cook for 5 minutes. To get 5-minutes cook time, "Pressure" button and use the Time Adjustment button to adjust the cook time to 5 minutes.

3. Pressure Release. Let the pressure to come down naturally for at least 15 minutes, then quick release any pressure left in the pot.

4. Finish the dish. Close crisping lid and select Broil, set time to 7 minutes. Remove from the pot. Perfect, juicy pork chops you may use the 'juice' in the pot to pour over the pork chops, or you can add a little polenta (or flour) and water, Sauté and make it like a gravy.

Serve and enjoy

Pork Chops With Applesauce

PREP: 10 MINUTES • PRESSURE: 10 MINUTES • AIR CRISP: 10 MINUTES • TOTAL: 30 MINUTES • PRESSURE LEVEL: HIGH • RELEASE: NATURAL
SERVES 2-4

Ingredients
2 – 4 pork loin chops (we used center cut, bone-on)
1 tablespoon grapeseed oil or olive oil
1 small onion, sliced

3 cloves garlic, roughly minced
2 gala apples, thinly sliced
2 pieces whole cloves (optional)
1 teaspoon cinnamon powder
1 tablespoon honey
½ cup unsalted homemade chicken stock or water
2 tablespoons light soy sauce
1 tablespoon butter
Kosher salt and ground black pepper to taste
1 ½ tablespoon cornstarch mixed with 2 tablespoons water (optional)

Directions
1. Preparing the Ingredients. Make a few small cut around the sides of the pork chops so they will stay flat and brown evenly.
Season the pork chops with a generous amount of kosher salt and ground black pepper.
Heat up your Multicooker. Add grapeseed oil into the pot. Add the seasoned pork chops into the pot, then let it brown for roughly 2 – 3 minutes on each side. Remove and set aside.
Add the sliced onions and stir. Add a pinch of kosher salt and ground black pepper to season if you like. Cook the onions for roughly 1 minute until softened. Then, add garlic and stir for 30 seconds until fragrance.
Add in the thinly sliced gala apples, whole cloves (optional) and cinnamon powder, then give it a quick stir. Add the honey and partially deglaze the bottom of the pot with a wooden spoon. Add chicken stock and light soy sauce, then fully deglaze the bottom of the pot with a wooden spoon. Taste the seasoning and add more salt and pepper if desired.
Place the pork chops back with all the meat juice into the pot.
2. High pressure for 10 minutes. Lock the lid on the Multicooker and then cook for 10 minutes. To get 10-minutes

cook time, press "Pressure" button and use the Time Adjustment button to adjust the cook time to 10 minutes.

3. Pressure Release. Let it fully natural release (roughly 10 minutes). Open the lid carefully.

4. Finish the dish. Close crisping lid. Select AIR CRISP, set temperature to 375°F, and set time to 10 minutes. Check after 10 minutes, cooking for an additional 5 minutes if dish needs more browning.

Remove the pork chops and set aside. Turn the Multicooker to the Sauté setting. Remove the cloves and taste the seasoning one more time. Add more salt and pepper if desired. Add butter and stir until it has fully dissolved into the sauce.

Mix the cornstarch with water and mix it into the applesauce one third at a time until desired thickness.

Drizzle the applesauce over the pork chops and serve immediately with side dishes.

Spare Ribs With Wine

PREP: 5 MINUTES • PRESSURE: 15 MINUTES • AIR CRISP: 10 MINUTES • TOTAL: 30 MINUTES • PRESSURE LEVEL: HIGH • RELEASE: NATURAL
SERVES 2-4

Ingredients
1 pound pork spare ribs, cut into pieces
1 tablespoon oil
1 tablespoon corn starch
1 – 2 teaspoon water
Green onions as garnish
1 teaspoon fish sauce (optional)
Black Bean Marinade:
1 tablespoon black bean sauce
1 tablespoon light soy sauce
1 tablespoon Shaoxing wine

1 tablespoon ginger, grated
3 cloves garlic, minced
1 teaspoon sesame oil
1 teaspoon sugar
A pinch of white pepper

Directions
1. Preparing the Ingredients. Marinate the pork spare ribs with Black Bean Marinade in an oven-safe bowl. Then, sit it in the fridge for 25 minutes.
First, mix 1 tablespoon of oil into the marinated spare ribs. Then, add 1 tablespoon of cornstarch and mix well. Finally, add 1 – 2 teaspoon of water into the spare ribs and mix well.
Add 1 cup of water into the Multicooker. Place steam rack in the Multicooker. Then, put the bowl of spare ribs on the rack.
2. High pressure for 15 minutes. Lock the lid on the Multicooker and then cook for 15 minutes. To get 15-minutes cook time, press "Pressure" Button and then adjust the time.
3. Pressure Release. Let the pressure to come down naturally for at least 15 minutes, then quick release any pressure left in the pot.
4. Finish the dish. Close crisping lid. Select AIR CRISP, set temperature to 375°F, and set time to 10 minutes. Check after 5 minutes, cooking for an additional 5 minutes if dish needs more browning.
Taste and add one teaspoon of fish sauce and green onions as garnish if you like.
Serve immediately.

Pork Loin With Apples

PREP: 5 MINUTES • PRESSURE: 30 MINUTES • TOTAL: 42 MINUTES • PRESSURE LEVEL: HIGH • RELEASE: QUICK SERVES 6-8

Ingredients

2 tablespoons unsalted butter
One 3-pound boneless pork loin roast
1 large red onion, halved and thinly sliced
2 medium tart green apples, such as Granny Smith, peeled, cored, and thinly sliced
4 fresh thyme sprigs
2 bay leaves
½ cup moderately sweet white wine, such as Riesling
¼ cup chicken broth
½ teaspoon salt
½ teaspoon ground black pepper

Directions

1. Preparing the Ingredients. Melt the butter in the Multicooker, set on the "Sauté" function. Add the pork loin and brown it on all sides, turning occasionally, about 8 minutes in all. Transfer to a large plate.

Add the onion to the pot; cook, often stirring, until softened, about 3 minutes. Stir in the apple, thyme, and bay leaves. Pour in the wine and scrape up any browned bits on the bottom of the pot.

Pour in the broth; stir in the salt and pepper. Nestle the pork loin into this apple mixture; pour any juices from the plate into the pot.

2. High pressure for 30 minutes. Lock the lid on the Multicooker and then cook for 30 minutes. To get 30-minutes cook time, press "Pressure" button and adjust the time.

3. Pressure Release. Use the quick-release method to bring the pot's pressure to normal.

4. Finish the dish. Close crisping lid and select Broil, set time to 7 minutes.

Transfer the pork to a cutting board; let stand for 5 minutes while you dish the sauce into serving bowls or onto a serving platter. Slice the loin into ½-inch-thick rounds and lay these over the sauce.

Pork Tenderloin And Coconut Rice

PREP: 5 MINUTES • PRESSURE: 15 MINUTES • TOTAL: 27 MINUTES • PRESSURE LEVEL: HIGH • RELEASE: QUICK SERVES 4

Ingredients
2 tablespoons peanut oil
1 pound pork tenderloin, cut into 4 pieces
1 small leek, white and pale green parts only, halved lengthwise, washed and thinly sliced
One 4½-ounce can chopped mild green chiles (about ½ cup)
1 teaspoon dried thyme
1 teaspoon ground cumin
½ teaspoon ground coriander
¼ teaspoon salt
¼ teaspoon ground black pepper
One 15-ounce can black beans, drained and rinsed (about 1¾ cups)
1 cup chicken broth
1 cup regular or low-fat canned coconut milk
1 cup white long-grain rice, such as white basmati rice
2 tablespoons packed light brown sugar

Directions

1. Preparing the Ingredients. Heat the oil in the Multicooker turned to the "Sauté" function. Add the pork tenderloin pieces; brown on all sides, occasionally turning, about 6 minutes. Transfer to a plate.

Add the leek and chiles; cook, often stirring, until the leek softens, about 2 minutes. Stir in the thyme, cumin, coriander, salt, and pepper; cook until aromatic, less than half a minute.

Stir in the beans, broth, coconut milk, rice, and brown sugar until the brown sugar dissolves.

Nestle the pieces of pork in the sauce, submerging the meat and rice as much as possible in the liquid; pour any juices from the meat's plate into the cooker.

2. High pressure for 15 minutes. Lock the lid on the Multicooker and then cook for 15 minutes. To get 15-minutes cook time, press "Pressure" Button and then adjust the time.

3. Pressure Release. Use the quick-release method to bring the pot's pressure back to normal but do not open the cooker. Set the pot aside for 10 minutes to steam the rice.

4. Finish the dish. Close crisping lid and select Broil, set time to 7 minutes.

Transfer the pork pieces to four serving plates; spoon the rice and beans around them.

Pork Tenderloin with Braised Apples
PREP: 5 MINUTES • PRESSURE: 45 MINUTES • TOTAL: 50 MINUTES • PRESSURE LEVEL: HIGH • RELEASE: QUICK
SERVES 4

Ingredients.
For The Brine (optional)
½ cup Diamond Crystal kosher salt, or ¼ cup fine table salt

¼ cup granulated sugar
2 cups very hot tap water
2 cups ice water

For The Pork And Apples
1 (1-pound) pork tenderloin, trimmed of silver skin and halved crosswise
Kosher salt, for salting and seasoning
2 tablespoons unsalted butter
1 cup thinly sliced onion
1 medium Granny Smith apple, or another tart apple, peeled and cut into ¼-inch slices
¾ cup apple juice, cider, or hard cider
½ cup low-sodium chicken broth
2 tablespoons heavy (whipping) cream
1 teaspoon Dijon mustard, plus additional as needed

Directions
1.   Preparing the Ingredients.
-To make the brine (if using)
In a large stainless steel or glass bowl, dissolve the salt and sugar in hot water; then stir in the ice water. Submerge the pork in the brine, and refrigerate for 2 to 3 hours. Drain and pat dry.
-To make the pork and apples
If you choose not to brine the pork, sprinkle it liberally with kosher salt.
Set to "Sauté/browning" heat the butter just until it stops foaming. Add the pork halves, browning on all sides, about 4 minutes total. Transfer to a plate or rack, and set aside.
Add the onion slices to the cooker, and cook, stirring, for 2 to 3 minutes, or until they just start to brown. Add the apple slices, and cook for 1 minute. Add the apple juice, and scrape the browned bits from the bottom of the pot. Bring to a simmer, and cook for 2 to 3 minutes, or until the juice has reduced by about one-third. Add the chicken broth, and return the pork tenderloin

to the cooker, placing the pieces on top of the apples and onions.

2. High pressure for 45 minutes. Lock the lid on the Multicooker and then cook for 45 minutes. To get 45-minutes cook time, press "Pressure" button and use the adjust button to adjust the cook time to 45 minutes.

3. Pressure Release. Use the quick-release method.

4. Finish the dish. Close crisping lid. Discard the bay leaves. Select AIR CRISP, set temperature to 375°F, and set time to 10 minutes. Check after 5 minutes, cooking for an additional 5 minutes if dish needs more browning.

Transfer the pork to a plate or rack, and tent it with aluminum foil while you finish the sauce.

Turn the Multicooker to "Sauté", simmer for about 6 minutes, or until the liquid is reduced by about half. Stir in the heavy cream and mustard, and taste, adding kosher salt or more mustard as needed.

Slice the pork into ¾-inch pieces, and place on a serving platter. Spoon the apples, onions, and sauce over the pork, and serve.

PER SERVING: CALORIES: 321; FAT: 13G; SODIUM: 754MG; CARBOHYDRATES: 21G; FIBER: 2G; PROTEIN: 32G

Pork Wonton Wonderful

PREP: 10 MINUTES • COOK TIME: 25 MINUTES • TOTAL: 35 MINUTES
SERVES: 3

Ingredients
- 8 wanton wrappers (Leasa brand works great, though any will do)
- 4 ounces of raw minced pork
- 1 medium-sized green apple
- 1 cup of water, for wetting the wanton wrappers
- 1 tablespoon of vegetable oil
- ½ tablespoon of oyster sauce
- 1 tablespoon of soy sauce
- Large pinch of ground white pepper

Directions:

1. Preparing the Ingredients. Cover the basket of the Crisplid-Pot with a lining of tin foil, leaving the edges uncovered to allow air to circulate through the basket. Preheat the Crisplid-Pot to 350 degrees.

In a small mixing bowl, combine the oyster sauce, soy sauce, and white pepper, then add in the minced pork and stir thoroughly. Cover and set in the fridge to marinate for at least 15 minutes. Core the apple, and slice into small cubes – smaller than bite-sized chunks.

Add the apples to the marinating meat mixture, and combine thoroughly. Spread the wonton wrappers, and fill each with a large spoonful of the filling. Wrap the wontons into triangles, so that the wrappers fully cover the filling, and seal with a drop of the water.

Coat each filled and wrapped wonton thoroughly with the vegetable oil, to help ensure a nice crispy fry. Place the wontons on the foil-lined air-fryer basket.

2. Air Frying. Set the Crisplid-Pot timer to 25 minutes. Halfway through cooking time, shake the handle of the Crisplid-Pot basket vigorously to jostle the wontons and ensure even frying. After 25 minutes, when the Crisplid-Pot shuts off, the wontons will be crispy golden-brown on the outside and juicy and delicious on the inside. Serve directly from the Crisplid-Pot basket and enjoy while hot.

Crispy Breaded Pork Chops

PREP: 10 MINUTES • COOK TIME: 15 MINUTES • TOTAL: 25 MINUTES
SERVES: 8

Ingredients
- 1/8 tsp. pepper
- ¼ tsp. chili powder
- ½ tsp. onion powder
- ½ tsp. garlic powder
- 1 ¼ tsp. sweet paprika
- 2 tbsp. grated parmesan cheese
- 1/3 C. crushed cornflake crumbs
- ½ C. panko breadcrumbs
- 1 beaten egg
- 6 center-cut boneless pork chops

Directions:

1 Preparing the Ingredients. Ensure that your Crisplid-Pot is preheated to 400 degrees. Spray the basket with olive oil.
With ½ teaspoon salt and pepper, season both sides of pork chops.

Combine ¾ teaspoon salt with pepper, chili powder, onion powder, garlic powder, paprika, cornflake crumbs, panko breadcrumbs, and parmesan cheese.
Beat egg in another bowl.
Dip pork chops into the egg and then crumb mixture.
Add pork chops to Crisplid-Pot and spritz with olive oil.

2   Air Frying. Set temperature to 400°F, and set time to 12 minutes. Cook 12 minutes, making sure to flip over halfway through the cooking process.

Only add 3 chops in at a time and repeat the process with remaining pork chops.

PER SERVING: CALORIES: 378; FAT: 13G; PROTEIN:33G; SUGAR:1

Roasted Pork Tenderloin

PREP: 5 MINUTES • COOK TIME: 1 HOUR • TOTAL: 65 MINUTES
SERVES: 4

Ingredients
  1 (3-pound) pork tenderloin
  2 tablespoons extra-virgin olive oil
  2 garlic cloves, minced
  1 teaspoon dried basil
  1 teaspoon dried oregano
  1 teaspoon dried thyme
  Salt
  Pepper

Directions:
1   Preparing the Ingredients. Drizzle the pork tenderloin with the olive oil.
Rub the garlic, basil, oregano, thyme, and salt and pepper to taste all over the tenderloin.

2   Air Frying. Place the tenderloin in the Crisplid-Pot. Cook for 45 minutes.
Use a meat thermometer to test for doneness
Open the Crisplid-Pot and flip the pork tenderloin. Cook for an additional 15 minutes.
Remove the cooked pork from the Crisplid-Pot and allow it to rest for 10 minutes before cutting.

PER SERVING: CALORIES: 283; FAT: 10G; PROTEIN:48

Bacon Wrapped Pork Tenderloin

PREP: 5 MINUTES • COOK TIME: 15 MINUTES • TOTAL: 20 MINUTES
SERVES: 4

Ingredients

Pork:
1-2 tbsp. Dijon mustard
3-4 strips of bacon
1 pork tenderloin
Apple Gravy:
½ - 1 tsp. Dijon mustard
1 tbsp. almond flour
2 tbsp. ghee
1 chopped onion
2-3 Granny Smith apples
1 C. vegetable broth

Directions:

1   Preparing the Ingredients. Spread Dijon mustard all over tenderloin and wrap the meat with strips of bacon.

2   Air Frying. Place into the Crisplid-Pot, set temperature to 360°F, and set time to 15 minutes and cook 10-15 minutes at 360 degrees. Use a meat thermometer to check for doneness.
To make sauce, heat ghee in a pan and add shallots. Cook 1-2 minutes.
Then add apples, cooking 3-5 minutes until softened.
Add flour and ghee to make a roux. Add broth and mustard, stirring well to combine.
When the sauce starts to bubble, add 1 cup of sautéed apples, cooking till sauce thickens.
Once pork tenderloin I cook, allow to sit 5-10 minutes to rest before slicing.
Serve topped with apple gravy.

PER SERVING: CALORIES: 552; FAT: 25G; PROTEIN:29G; SUGAR:6G

Dijon Garlic Pork Tenderloin
PREP: 5 MINUTES • COOK TIME: 10 MINUTES • TOTAL: 15 MINUTES
SERVES: 6

Ingredients
    1 C. breadcrumbs
    Pinch of cayenne pepper
    3 crushed garlic cloves
    2 tbsp. ground ginger
    2 tbsp. Dijon mustard
    2 tbsp. raw honey
    4 tbsp. water
    2 tsp. salt
    1 pound pork tenderloin, sliced into 1-inch rounds

Directions:

1. Preparing the Ingredients. With pepper and salt, season all sides of tenderloin.

Combine cayenne pepper, garlic, ginger, mustard, honey, and water until smooth.

Dip pork rounds into the honey mixture and then into breadcrumbs, ensuring they all get coated well.

Place coated pork rounds into your Crisplid-Pot.

2. Air Frying. Set temperature to 400°F, and set time to 10 minutes. Cook 10 minutes at 400 degrees. Flip and then cook an additional 5 minutes until golden in color.

PER SERVING: CALORIES: 423; FAT: 18G; PROTEIN:31G; SUGAR:3G

Chinese Braised Pork Belly

PREP: 5 MINUTES • COOK TIME: 20 MINUTES • TOTAL: 25 MINUTES
SERVES: 8

Ingredients
- 1 lb Pork Belly, sliced
- 1 Tbsp Oyster Sauce
- 1 Tbsp Sugar
- 2 Red Fermented Bean Curds
- 1 Tbsp Red Fermented Bean Curd Paste
- 1 Tbsp Cooking Wine
- 1/2 Tbsp Soy Sauce
- 1 Tsp Sesame Oil
- 1 Cup All Purpose Flour

Directions:

1   Preparing the Ingredients. Preheat the Crisplid-Pot to 390 degrees.

In a small bowl, mix all ingredients together and rub the pork thoroughly with this mixture

Set aside to marinate for at least 30 minutes or preferably overnight for the flavors to permeate the meat

Coat each marinated pork belly slice in flour and place in the Crisplid-Pot tray

2   Air Frying. Cook for 15 to 20 minutes until crispy and tender.

Air Fryer Sweet and Sour Pork

PREP: 10 MINUTES • COOK TIME: 12 MINUTES • TOTAL: 22 MINUTES
SERVES: 6

Ingredients
- 3 tbsp. olive oil
- 1/16 tsp. Chinese Five Spice
- ¼ tsp. pepper
- ½ tsp. sea salt
- 1 tsp. pure sesame oil
- 2 eggs
- 1 C. almond flour
- 2 pounds pork, sliced into chunks

Sweet and Sour Sauce:
- ¼ tsp. sea salt
- ½ tsp. garlic powder
- 1 tbsp. low-sodium soy sauce
- ½ C. rice vinegar
- 5 tbsp. tomato paste
- 1/8 tsp. water
- ½ C. sweetener of choice

Directions:

1   Preparing the Ingredients. To make the dipping sauce, whisk all sauce ingredients together over medium heat, stirring 5 minutes. Simmer uncovered 5 minutes till thickened.

Meanwhile, combine almond flour, five spice, pepper, and salt. In another bowl, mix eggs with sesame oil.

Dredge pork in flour mixture and then in egg mixture. Shake any excess off before adding to Crisplid-Pot basket.

2   Air Frying. Set temperature to 340°F, and set time to 12 minutes.

Serve with sweet and sour dipping sauce!

PER SERVING: CALORIES: 371; FAT: 17G; PROTEIN:27G; SUGAR:1G

Fried Pork Scotch Egg

PREP: 10 MINUTES • COOK TIME: 25 MINUTES • TOTAL: 35 MINUTES
SERVES: 2

Ingredients
   3 soft-boiled eggs, peeled
   8 ounces of raw minced pork, or sausage outside the casings
   2 teaspoons of ground rosemary
   2 teaspoons of garlic powder
   Pinch of salt and pepper
   2 raw eggs
   1 cup of breadcrumbs (Panko, but other brands are fine, or home-made bread crumbs work too)

Directions:

1.   Preparing the Ingredients. Cover the basket of the Crisplid-Pot with a lining of tin foil, leaving the edges uncovered to allow air to circulate through the basket. Preheat the Crisplid-Pot to 350 degrees.
In a mixing bowl, combine the raw pork with the rosemary, garlic powder, salt, and pepper. This will probably be easiest to do with your masher or bare hands (though make sure to wash thoroughly after handling raw meat!); combine until all the spices are evenly spread throughout the meat.
Divide the meat mixture into three equal portions in the mixing bowl, and form each into balls with your hands.
Lay a large sheet of plastic wrap on the countertop, and flatten one of the balls of meat on top of it, to form a wide, flat meat-circle.

Place one of the peeled soft-boiled eggs in the center of the meat-circle and then, using the ends of the plastic wrap, pull the meat-circle so that it is fully covering and surrounding the soft-boiled egg.

Tighten and shape the plastic wrap covering the meat so that if forms a ball, and make sure not to squeeze too hard lest you squish the soft-boiled egg at the center of the ball! Set aside.

Repeat steps 5-7 with the other two soft-boiled eggs and portions of meat-mixture.

In a separate mixing bowl, beat the two raw eggs until fluffy and until the yolks and whites are fully combined.

One by one, remove the plastic wrap and dunk the pork-covered balls into the raw egg, and then roll them in the bread crumbs, covering fully and generously.

Place each of the bread-crumb covered meat-wrapped balls onto the foil-lined surface of the Crisplid-Pot. Three of them should fit nicely, without touching.

2.   Air Frying. Set the Crisplid-Pot timer to 25 minutes. About halfway through the cooking time, shake the handle of the air-fryer vigorously, so that the scotch eggs inside roll around and ensure full coverage.

After 25 minutes, the Crisplid-Pot will shut off, and the scotch eggs should be perfect – the meat fully cooked, the egg-yolks still runny on the inside, and the outsides crispy and golden-brown. Using tongs, place them on serving plates, slice in half, and enjoy

Teriyaki Pork Rolls

PREP: 10 MINUTES • COOK TIME: 8 MINUTES • TOTAL: 20 MINUTES
SERVES: 6

Ingredients
- 1 tsp. almond flour
- 4 tbsp. low-sodium soy sauce

4 tbsp. mirin
4 tbsp. brown sugar
Thumb-sized amount of ginger, chopped
Pork belly slices
Enoki mushrooms

Directions:

1. Preparing the Ingredients. Mix brown sugar, mirin, soy sauce, almond flour, and ginger together until brown sugar dissolves.

Take pork belly slices and wrap around a bundle of mushrooms. Brush each roll with teriyaki sauce. Chill half an hour. Preheat your Crisplid-Pot to 350 degrees and add marinated pork rolls.

2. Air Frying. Set temperature to 350°F, and set time to 8 minutes.

PER SERVING: CALORIES: 412; FAT: 9G; PROTEIN:19G; SUGAR:4G

Beef Recipes

Classic Pot Roast

PREP: 5 MINUTES • PRESSURE: 90 MINUTES • BROIL: 8 MINUTES • TOTAL: 103 MINUTES • PRESSURE LEVEL: HIGH • RELEASE: QUICK AND NATURAL
SERVES: 6

Ingredients
1 tablespoon olive oil
One 3- to 3½-pound boneless beef chuck roast
1 teaspoon salt
½ teaspoon ground black pepper
1 large yellow onion, chopped
2 teaspoons minced garlic
Up to 1½ cups beef broth
3 tablespoons tomato paste
One 4-inch rosemary sprig
½ ounce dried mushrooms, preferably porcini
1½ pounds small white or yellow potatoes

Directions
1. Preparing the Ingredients. Heat the oil in the Multicooker. Turn on the Multicooker to the Sauté setting then wait for it to boil.
Season the roast with the salt and pepper; brown it on both sides, turning once, about 10 minutes. Transfer the meat to a large bowl.
Add the onion; cook, often stirring, until translucent, about 4 minutes. Add the garlic; cook, stirring constantly, until aromatic, about 30 seconds. Pour 1¼ cup broth in the Multicooker. Add the tomato paste and stir well until dissolved. Tuck the rosemary

into the sauce and crumble in the mushrooms. Nestle the meat into the sauce, adding any juices in the bowl.
2. High pressure for 60 minutes. Close the lid and the pressure valve and then cook for 60 minutes. To get 60-minutes cook time, press "Pressure" button and use the Time Adjustment button to adjust the cook time to 60 minutes.
3. Pressure Release. Use the quick-release method.
Unlock and open the cooker; sprinkle the potatoes around the meat.
4. High pressure for 30 minutes. Close the lid and the pressure valve again and cook for 30 minutes. To get 30-minutes cook time, press "Pressure" button.
5. Pressure Release. Use the natural-release method -20 to 30 minutes.
6. Finish the dish. Close crisping lid. Select BROIL, and set time to 8 minutes. Check after 5 minutes, cooking for an additional 3 minutes if dish needs more browning.
Transfer the roast to a cutting board; set aside for 5 minutes. Discard the rosemary sprig. Slice the meat into 2-inch irregular chunks and serve these in bowls with the vegetables, mushrooms, and broth.
Serve and Enjoy!

Spicy Thai Beef Stir-Fry

PREP: 15 MINUTES • COOK TIME: 9 MINUTES • TOTAL: 24 MINUTES
SERVES: 4

Ingredients
   1 pound sirloin steaks, thinly sliced
   2 tablespoons lime juice, divided
   ⅓ cup crunchy peanut butter
   ½ cup beef broth
   1 tablespoon olive oil

1½ cups broccoli florets
2 cloves garlic, sliced
1 to 2 red chile peppers, sliced

Directions:

1   Preparing the Ingredients. In a medium bowl, combine the steak with 1 tablespoon of the lime juice. Set aside.

Combine the peanut butter and beef broth in a small bowl and mix well. Drain the beef and add the juice from the bowl into the peanut butter mixture.

In a 6-inch metal bowl, combine the olive oil, steak, and broccoli.

2   Air Frying. Cook for 3 to 4 minutes or until the steak is almost cooked and the broccoli is crisp and tender, shaking the basket once during cooking time.

Add the garlic, chile peppers, and the peanut butter mixture and stir.

Cook for 3 to 5 minutes or until the sauce is bubbling and the broccoli is tender.

Serve over hot rice.

PER SERVING: CALORIES: 387; FAT: 22G; PROTEIN:42G; FIBER:2G

Brisket With Veggies

PREP: 10 MINUTES • PRESSURE: 60 MINUTES • BROIL: 8 MINUTES • TOTAL: 78 MINUTES • PRESSURE LEVEL: HIGH • RELEASE: QUICK
SERVES 6

Ingredients
2 tbs. olive oil
5 or 6 red potatoes
2 lb. or larger regular brisket, rinsed and patted dry

Fresh ground black pepper
3 tbs. heaping chopped garlic
1 lg. yellow onion
2 c. large chunks carrots
2-½ c. homemade beef broth, or make from Knorr Beef Base
3 tbs. Worcestershire Sauce
4 bay leaves
5 or 6 red potatoes
Granulated garlic
Knorr Demi-Glace sauce
½ c. dehydrated onion
2 stalks celery in 1" chunks

Directions
1. Preparing the Ingredients. Put the Multicooker on the sauté setting.
Put in 1 tbs. (more if needed) of the oil and caramelize the onions. Once golden, remove from pot, put in a bowl, and set aside. But keep the Multicooker on the "Sauté" setting.
Rub the freshly ground pepper on both sides of the brisket. Do the same with the granulated garlic. Add 1tbs. olive oil (or more) and only lightly sear the brisket on all sides.
Add back the onions, garlic, Worcestershire sauce, bay leaves, dehydrated onion and beef broth.
2. High pressure for 50 minutes. Close the lid and the pressure valve and then cook for 50 minutes. To get 50-minutes cook time, press "Pressure" button and use the Time Adjustment button to adjust the cook time to 50 minutes.
While the meat is cooking, peel and cut up all the veggies. When the meat is done, use the quick pressure release feature, and then remove the lid. Add all of the veggies, replace the lid and cook at high pressure for to 10 minutes. To get 10-minutes cook time, press "Steam" button
3. Pressure Release. When the time is up, turn the pot off, use the quick release again, and remove the lid.

4. Finish the dish. Close crisping lid. Select BROIL, and set time to 8 minutes. Check after 5 minutes, cooking for an additional 3 minutes if dish needs more browning.
Use a platter to remove the veggies and meat. Use the "Sauté" setting and bring the broth to a boil, then add the Knorr Demi-Glace mixing with a Wisk. Adjust seasonings as needed. Serve with Cole Slaw or other salad, homemade rolls or Italian garlic bread. Be sure to remove the bay leaves before serving.
Serve and Enjoy

Per Serving Calories: 425; Total Carbohydrates: 50g; Saturated Fat: 3.6g; Trans Fat: 0g; Fiber: 10.6g; Protein: 30.5g; Sodium: 490mg

Steak and Mushroom Gravy
PREP: 15 MINUTES • COOK TIME: 15 MINUTES • TOTAL: 30 MINUTES
SERVES: 4

Ingredients
- 4 cubed steaks
- 2 large eggs
- 1/2 dozen mushrooms
- 4 tablespoons unsalted butter
- 4 tablespoons black pepper
- 2 tablespoons salt
- 1/2 teaspoon onion powder
- 1/2 teaspoon garlic powder
- 1/4 teaspoon cayenne powder
- 1 1/4 teaspoons paprika
- 1 1/2 cups whole milk
- 1/3 cup flour
- 2 tablespoons vegetable oil

Directions:

1   Preparing the Ingredients. Mix 1/2 flour and a pinch of black pepper in a shallow bowl or on a plate.

Beat 2 eggs in a bowl and mix in a pinch of salt and pepper.

In another shallow bowl mix together the other half of the flour with a pepper to taste, garlic powder, paprika, cayenne, and onion powder.

Chop mushrooms and set aside.

Press your steak into the first flour bowl, then dip in egg, then press the steak into the second flour bowl until covered completely.

2   Air Frying. Cook steak at 360 degrees for 15 Minutes, flipping halfway through.

While the steak cooks, warm the butter over medium heat and add mushrooms to sauté.

Add 4 tablespoons of the flour and pepper mix to the pan and mix until there are no clumps of flour.

Mix in whole milk and simmer.

Serve over steak for breakfast, lunch, or dinner.

PER SERVING: CALORIES: 442; FAT: 27G; PROTEIN:32G; FIBER:2.3G

Korean Braised Short Ribs

PREP: 10 MINUTES • PRESSURE: 45 MINUTES • BROIL: 8 MINUTES • TOTAL: 63 MINUTES • PRESSURE LEVEL: HIGH • RELEASE: NATURAL

SERVES 4-6

Ingredients
1 teaspoon vegetable oil
2 green onions cut into 1-inch lengths
3 cloves garlic, smashed
3 quarter-sized slices of ginger
4 pounds beef short ribs, about 3 inches thick, cut into 3 rib portions
1/2-cup water
1/2-cup soy sauce
1/4-cup rice wine (or dry sherry)
1/4-cup pear juice (or apple juice)
2 teaspoons sesame oil
Minced green onions
Gochujang sauce

Directions
1. Preparing the Ingredients. Heat the vegetable oil in the Multicooker using the "Sauté" function, until the oil is shimmering. Add the green onion, garlic, and ginger, and sauté for 1 minute, or until you can smell the garlic. Add the short ribs, water, soy sauce, rice wine, pear juice and sesame oil. Stir until the ribs are completely coated.
2. High pressure for 45 minutes. Lock the lid on the Multicooker and then cook for 45 minutes. To get 45-minutes cook time, press Meat/Chicken button and use the ADJUST button to adjust the cook time to 45 minutes.
3. Pressure Release. Let the pressure to come down naturally for at least 15 minutes, then quick release any pressure left in the pot.
4. Finish the dish. Close crisping lid. Select BROIL, and set time to 8 minutes. Check after 5 minutes, cooking for an additional 3 minutes if dish needs more browning.
Remove the short ribs from the pot with a slotted spoon.
Serve the ribs with the degreased sauce.

Meat Lovers' Pizza

PREP: 10 MINUTES • COOK TIME: 12 MINUTES • TOTAL: 22 MINUTES
SERVES: 2

Ingredients

- 1 pre-prepared 7-inch pizza pie crust, defrosted if necessary.
- 1/3 cup of marinara sauce.
- 2 ounces of grilled steak, sliced into bite-sized pieces
- 2 ounces of salami, sliced fine
- 2 ounces of pepperoni, sliced fine
- ¼ cup of American cheese
- ¼ cup of shredded mozzarella cheese

Directions:

1. Preparing the Ingredients. Preheat the Crisplid-Pot to 350 degrees. Lay the pizza dough flat on a sheet of parchment paper or tin foil, cut large enough to hold the entire pie crust, but small enough that it will leave the edges of the air frying basket uncovered to allow for air circulation. Using a fork, stab the pizza dough several times across the surface – piercing the pie crust will allow air to circulate throughout the crust and ensure even cooking. With a deep soup spoon, ladle the marinara sauce onto the pizza dough, and spread evenly in expanding circles over the surface of the pie-crust. Be sure to leave at least ½ inch of bare dough around the edges, to ensure that extra-crispy crunchy first bite of the crust! Distribute the pieces of steak and the slices of salami and pepperoni evenly over the sauce-covered dough, then sprinkle the cheese in an even layer on top.
2. Air Frying. Set the Crisplid-Pot timer to 12 minutes, and place the pizza with foil or paper on the fryer's basket surface. Again, be sure to leave the edges of the basket

uncovered to allow for proper air circulation, and don't let your bare fingers touch the hot surface. After 12 minutes, when the Crisplid-Pot shuts off, the cheese should be perfectly melted and lightly crisped, and the pie crust should be golden brown. Using a spatula – or two, if necessary, remove the pizza from the Crisplid-Pot basket and set on a serving plate. Wait a few minutes until the pie is cool enough to handle, then cut into slices and serve.

Thai Red Beef Curry

PREP: 15 MINUTES • PRESSURE: 45 MINUTES • BROIL: 8 MINUTES • TOTAL: 68 MINUTES • PRESSURE LEVEL: MEDIUM • RELEASE: NATURAL

SERVES 6-8

Ingredients

1 tablespoon vegetable oil
1 medium onion, peeled and sliced into 1/2 inch wedges
1 red bell pepper, cored, stemmed, and sliced into 1/2 inch strips
3 cloves garlic, crushed
1/2 inch piece of ginger, peeled and crushed
Cream from the top of a (13.5 ounce) can coconut milk
4 tablespoons red curry paste (a whole 4 oz. can)
8-ounce can bamboo shoots, drained
2 pounds flat iron steak (or chuck blade steak), cut into 2 inches by 1/2 inch strips
1 teaspoon Diamond Crystal kosher salt or 2 teaspoons fine sea salt
1/2 cup chicken stock or water
1 tablespoon fish sauce (plus more to taste)
1 tablespoon soy sauce (plus more to taste)
Juice of 1 lime
Minced cilantro
Minced basil (preferably Thai basil)

Lime wedges
Jasmine rice

Directions

1. Preparing the Ingredients. Heat the vegetable oil in the Multicooker using the "Sauté" function, until the oil is shimmering. Stir in the onion, red bell pepper, garlic, and ginger, and sauté until the onion starts to soften about 3 minutes.

Fry the curry paste: Scoop the cream from the top of the can of coconut milk and add it to the pot, then stir in the curry paste. Cook, often stirring, until the curry paste darkens, about 5 minutes.

Sprinkle the beef with the kosher salt. Add the beef to the pot, and stir to coat with curry paste. Stir in the rest of the can of coconut milk, bamboo shoots, chicken stock, fish sauce, and soy sauce.

2. High pressure for 12 minutes. Lock the lid on the Multicooker and then cook for 12 minutes. To get 12-minutes cook time, press "Pressure" button and adjust the cook time.

3. Pressure Release. Let the pressure to come down naturally for at least 20 minutes, then quick release any pressure left in the pot.

4. Finish the dish. Remove the lid from the Multicooker. Close crisping lid. Select BROIL, and set time to 8 minutes. Check after 5 minutes, cooking for an additional 3 minutes if dish needs more browning.

Stir in the limejuice, and then taste the curry for seasoning, adding more fish sauce or brown sugar as needed. Ladle the curry into bowls, sprinkle with minced cilantro and basil, and serve with Jasmine rice.

Serve and Enjoy

Per Serving Calories: 321.5; Protein: 28.8g

Air Fryer Roast Beef

PREP: 5 MINUTES • COOK TIME: 45 MINUTES • TOTAL: 50 MINUTES
SERVES: 6

Ingredients
Roast beef
1 tbsp. olive oil
Seasonings of choice

Directions:
1   Preparing the Ingredients. Ensure your Crisplid-Pot is preheated to 160 degrees.
Place roast in bowl and toss with olive oil and desired seasonings.
Put seasoned roast into the Crisplid-Pot.
2   Air Frying. Set temperature to 160°F, and set time to 30 minutes and cook 30 minutes.
Turn roast when the timer sounds and cook another 15 minutes.

PER SERVING: CALORIES: 267; FAT: 8G; PROTEIN:2G

Beef Ribs

PREP: 10 MINUTES • PRESSURE: 60 MINUTES • BROIL: 10 MINUTES • TOTAL: 80 MINUTES • PRESSURE LEVEL: HIGH • RELEASE: NORMAL
SERVES 4-6

Ingredients

1 tablespoon sesame oil
2 cloves garlic, peeled and smashed
1" knob fresh ginger, peeled and finely chopped
1 pinch red pepper flakes
¼ cup rice vinegar (or white balsamic vinegar)
⅓ cup raw sugar
⅔ cup soy sauce
⅔ cup salt-free (home made) beef stock
4 pounds (2k) beef ribs (about 8), ask the butcher to saw or chop them in half
2 tablespoons cornstarch
1-2 tablespoons water

Directions

1. Preparing the Ingredients. Turn on the Multicooker to "Sauté" mode.
Add sesame oil garlic, ginger and red pepper flakes and sauté for a minute.
Then, de-glaze with vinegar, mix-in the sugar, soy sauce and beef stock - mix well.
Add the ribs to the Multicooker coating them with the mixture.
2. High pressure for 60 minutes. Close and lock the lid of the Multicooker, cook at high pressure for 60 minutes. To get 60-minutes cook time, press "Pressure" button and use the Time Adjustment button to adjust the cook time to 60 minutes.
3. Pressure Release. Use the Natural release method (20 minutes).
4. Finish the dish. Remove the lid from the Multicooker. Close crisping lid. Select BROIL, and set time to 10 minutes. Check after 6 minutes, cooking for an additional 4 minutes if dish needs more browning.

Make a slurry with the cornstarch and water and then mix into the rib cooking liquid in the Multicooker. "Sauté" the mixture until it reaches the desired consistency.
Serve and Enjoy!

Per Serving Calories: 307.3; Carbohydrates: 8.6g; Fat: 10.7g; Fiber: 10.6g; Protein: 32.3g; Sodium: 1654.6mg; Cholesterol: 89.2g

Crispy Mongolian Beef
PREP: 5 MINUTES • COOK TIME: 10 MINUTES • TOTAL: 15 MINUTES
SERVES: 6

Ingredients
- Olive oil
- ½ C. almond flour
- 2 pounds beef tenderloin or beef chuck, sliced into strips
- Sauce:
- ½ C. chopped green onion
- 1 tsp. red chili flakes
- 1 tsp. almond flour
- ½ C. brown sugar
- 1 tsp. hoisin sauce
- ½ C. water
- ½ C. rice vinegar
- ½ C. low-sodium soy sauce
- 1 tbsp. chopped garlic
- 1 tbsp. finely chopped ginger
- 2 tbsp. olive oil

Directions:
1. Preparing the Ingredients. Toss strips of beef in almond flour, ensuring they are coated well. Add to the Crisplid-Pot.

2. Air Frying. Set temperature to 300°F, and set time to 10 minutes, and cook 10 minutes at 300 degrees.

Meanwhile, add all sauce ingredients to the pan and bring to a boil. Mix well.

Add beef strips to the sauce and cook 2 minutes.

Serve over cauliflower rice!

PER SERVING: CALORIES: 290; FAT: 14G; PROTEIN:22G; SUGAR:1G

Lamb Casserole

PREP: 15 MINUTES • PRESSURE: 35 MINUTES • AIR CRISP: 15 MINUTES • TOTAL: 65 MINUTES • PRESSURE LEVEL: HIGH • RELEASE: NORMAL
SERVES 6-8

Ingredients
1 pound of baby potatoes
1 pound rack of lamb
2 carrots
1 large onion
2 stalks of celery
1-2 teaspoons of salt depending on the salt content of the chicken stock
2 medium size tomatoes
2 cups of chicken stock
3-4 large cloves of garlic
2 teaspoon of cumin powder
2 teaspoon of Paprika
A pinch of dried rosemary
A pinch of dried oregano leaves
2 tablespoons of ketchup
3 tablespoons of sherry or red wine

A splash of beer if you have one in hand

Directions
1. Preparing the Ingredients. Dice the tomatoes, onion, and garlic, cut potatoes, and carrots, cut the rack of lamb into two halves. Put all the ingredients, in the Multicooker.
2. High pressure for 35 minutes. Lock the lid on the Multicooker and then cook for 35 minutes. To get 35-minutes cook time, press "Pressure" button and adjust the time.
3. Pressure Release. Use Natural-Release Method for 10 minutes, and then Quick-Release.
4. Remove the lid from the Multicooker. Close crisping lid. Select AIR CRISP, set temperature to 400°F, and set time to 15 minutes. Check after 10 minutes, cooking for an additional 5 minutes if dish needs more browning.

Serve and Enjoy!

Per Serving Calories: 407.3; Carbohydrates: 6.6g; Fat: 11.7g; Fiber: 8.6g; Protein: 35.3g; Sodium: 1640.6mg; Cholesterol: 77.2

Swedish Meatballs

PREP: 10 MINUTES • COOK TIME: 14 MINUTES • TOTAL: 24 MINUTES
SERVES: 4

Ingredients
For the meatballs
- 1 pound 93% lean ground beef
- 1 (1-ounce) packet Lipton Onion Recipe Soup & Dip Mix
- ⅓ cup bread crumbs
- 1 egg, beaten
- Salt
- Pepper

For the gravy
- 1 cup beef broth
- ⅓ cup heavy cream
- 1 tablespoons all-purpose flour

Directions:

1. Preparing the Ingredients. In a large bowl, combine the ground beef, onion soup mix, bread crumbs, egg, and salt and pepper to taste. Mix thoroughly.

Using 2 tablespoons of the meat mixture, create each meatball by rolling the beef mixture around in your hands. This should yield about 10 meatballs.

2. Air Frying. Place the meatballs in the Crisplid-Pot. It is okay to stack them. Cook for 14 minutes.

While the meatballs cook, prepare the gravy. Heat a saucepan over medium-high heat.

Add the beef broth and heavy cream. Stir for 1 to 2 minutes.

Add the flour and stir. Cover and allow the sauce to simmer for 3 to 4 minutes, or until thick.

Drizzle the gravy over the meatballs and serve.

PER SERVING: CALORIES: 178; FAT: 14G; PROTEIN:9G; FIBER:0

Barbecued Baby Back Ribs

PREP: 5 MINUTES • PRESSURE: 32 MINUTES • AIR CRISP: 15 MINUTES • TOTAL: 52 MINUTES • PRESSURE LEVEL: HIGH • RELEASE: NATURAL
SERVES 4

Ingredients

¼ cup canned tomato paste
2 tablespoons cider vinegar
1 tablespoon sweet paprika
½ tablespoon coriander seeds
½ tablespoon fennel seeds
1 teaspoon onion powder
1 teaspoon dried thyme
½ teaspoon ground allspice
½ teaspoon salt
½ teaspoon ground black pepper
¼ teaspoon celery seeds
One 4-pound rack baby back ribs, cut into 2 or 3 sections to fit in the cooker

Directions

1. Preparing the Ingredients. Whisk the tomato paste, vinegar, paprika, coriander and fennel seeds, onion powder, thyme, allspice, salt, pepper, and celery seeds with ¾ cup water in an electric Multicooker until the tomato paste dissolves. Add the ribs; toss to coat thoroughly and evenly in the sauce.

2. High pressure for 32 minutes. Lock the lid on the Multicooker and then cook for 32 minutes. To get 32-minutes cook time, press "Pressure" button and use the Time Adjustment button to adjust the cook time to 32 minutes.

3. Pressure Release. Let the pressure to come down naturally for at least 15 minutes, then quick release any pressure left in the pot.

4. Finish the dish. Remove the lid from the Multicooker. Close crisping lid. Select AIR CRISP, set temperature to 400°F, and set time to 15 minutes. Check after 10 minutes, cooking for an additional 5 minutes if dish needs more browning.

5. Transfer the rib rack sections to a large rimmed baking sheet. Set the electric one to its browning function. Bring the sauce to a simmer. Cook, stirring occasionally, until the sauce has thickened, 3 to 5 minutes.

Position the oven rack 4 to 6 inches from the broiler; heat the broiler. Brush a light coating of the sauce onto the ribs, then broil until glazed and hot, 6 to 8 minutes, turning once. Slice the

Sausage And Peppers

PREP: 5 MINUTES • PRESSURE: 10 MINUTES • AIR CRISP: 10 MINUTES • TOTAL: 25 MINUTES • PRESSURE LEVEL: HIGH • RELEASE: QUICK
SERVES 6

Ingredients
2 tablespoons olive oil
2½ pounds sweet Italian sausages in their casings
4 large red bell peppers, stemmed, seeded, and cut into strips
1 medium red onion, halved and thinly sliced
2 medium garlic cloves, slivered
1 cup red (sweet) vermouth
2 tablespoons balsamic vinegar
¼ teaspoon grated nutmeg

Directions

1. Preparing the Ingredients. Heat the oil in a Multicooker, turned to the sauté function. Prick the sausages with a fork, add them to the pot, and brown on all sides, about 6 minutes. Transfer to a large bowl.

Add the peppers and onion; cook, stirring almost constantly, just until the pepper strips glisten, about 2 minutes. Add the garlic, cook a few seconds, and then stir in the vermouth, vinegar, and nutmeg. Nestle the sausages into the mixture.

2. High pressure for 10 minutes. Lock the lid on the Multicooker and Cook for 10 minutes. To get 10-minutes cook time, press the "Pressure" button and adjust the time.

3. Pressure Release. Use the quick-release method to bring the pot's pressure back to normal.

4. Remove the lid from the Multicooker. Close crisping lid. Select AIR CRISP, set temperature to 390°F, and set time to 10 minutes. Check after 8 minutes, cooking for an additional 2 minutes if dish needs more browning.

Stir well before serving.

Spicy Sausage And Chard Pasta Sauce
PREP: 5 MINUTES • PRESSURE: 6 MINUTES • BROIL: 5 MINUTES • TOTAL: 16 MINUTES • PRESSURE LEVEL: HIGH • RELEASE: QUICK
SERVES 6

Ingredients
2 tablespoons olive oil
1 medium red onion, chopped

Up to 3 small hot chiles, such as cherry peppers or Anaheim chiles, stemmed, seeded, and chopped
1 tablespoon minced garlic
1 pound mild Italian pork sausage meat, any casings removed
½ cup dry red wine, such as Syrah
½ cup canned tomato paste
¼ cup chicken broth
1 tablespoon dried basil
2 teaspoons dried oregano
4 cups stemmed and chopped Swiss chard

Directions
1.   Preparing the Ingredients. Heat the oil in a Multicooker, turned to the sauté function.
Add the onion and cook, often stirring, until softened, about 4 minutes. Add the chiles and garlic; cook until aromatic, stirring all the while, about 1 minute.
Crumble in the sausage meat, breaking up any clumps with a wooden spoon. Stir until it loses its raw color. Stir in the wine, tomato paste, broth, basil, and oregano until the tomato paste dissolves. Add the chard and stir well.
2.   High pressure for 6 minutes. Lock the lid onto the cooker, set the machine's timer to cook at high pressure for 6 minutes. To get 6-minutes cook time, press the "Pressure" button and use the Time Adjustment button to adjust the cook time to 6 minutes.
3.   Pressure Release. Use the quick-release method to drop the pressure back to normal.
4.   Finish the dish. Remove the lid from the Multicooker. Close crisping lid. Select BROIL, and set time to 5 minutes. Check after 4 minutes, cooking for an additional 4 minutes if dish needs more browning.
Stir well before serving.

Ground Beef Stew

PREP: 5 MINUTES • PRESSURE: 5 MINUTES • AIR CRISP: 15 MINUTES • TOTAL: 25 MINUTES • PRESSURE LEVEL: HIGH • RELEASE: QUICK
SERVES 4

Ingredients
1 tablespoon olive oil
1½ pounds lean ground beef (about 93% lean)
1 large yellow onion, chopped
1 large sweet potato (about 1 pound), peeled and shredded through the large holes of a box grater
1 teaspoon ground cinnamon
1 teaspoon ground cumin
½ teaspoon dried sage
½ teaspoon dried oregano
½ teaspoon salt
½ teaspoon ground black pepper
2 tablespoons yellow cornmeal
2 tablespoons honey
2½ cups beef broth

Directions
1. Preparing the Ingredients. Heat the oil in the Multicooker turned to the Sauté function. Crumble in the ground beef; cook, stirring occasionally, until it loses its raw color and browns a bit, about 5 minutes. Add the onion; cook, often stirring, until softened, about 3 minutes.
Stir in the sweet potato, cinnamon, cumin, sage, oregano, salt, and pepper. Cook for 1 minute, stirring constantly. Stir in the

cornmeal and honey; cook for 1 minute, often stirring, to dissolve the cornmeal. Stir in the broth.
2. High pressure for 5 minutes. Lock the lid on the Multicooker and then cook for 5 minutes. To get 5-minutes cook time, press "Pressure" button and use the Time Adjustment button to adjust the cook time to 5 minutes.
3. Pressure Release. Use the quick-release method to drop the pot's pressure to normal.
4. Finish the dish. Remove the lid from the Multicooker. Close crisping lid. Select AIR CRISP, set temperature to 390°F, and set time to 20 minutes. Check after 15 minutes, cooking for an additional 15 minutes if dish needs more browning.
Stir well and set aside, loosely covered, for 5 minutes before serving.

Lamb with Mexican Sauce

PREP: 10 MINUTES • PRESSURE: 45 MINUTES • AIR CRISP: 15 MINUTES • TOTAL: 70 MINUTES • PRESSURE LEVEL: HIGH • RELEASE: NORMAL
SERVES 3-4

Ingredients
3 lamb shoulder
1 Spanish onion
3 garlic cloves, minced
1 19 oz. can Old El Paso Enchilada sauce
2 Tbsp. oil
Salt to taste
Cilantro, chopped without the stems
Corn tortillas (3-4 per person)
Limes cut into 8ths
Black beans or refried beans
Chipotle-style rice

Directions
1. Preparing the Ingredients. Marinate lamb overnight in Old El Paso Enchilada sauce (mild, medium or hot).
Turn on the Multicooker to "sauté" mode.
Add oil. Put in the onions and cook until soft, add garlic and cook for 1 minute.
Add the lamb and marinade wait until boil.
2. High pressure for 45 minutes. Lock the lid on the Multicooker and then cook for 45 minutes. To get 45-minutes cook time, press "Pressure" button and use the adjust button to adjust the cook time to 45 minutes.
3. Pressure Release. Let the pressure to come down naturally for at least 15 minutes, then quick release any pressure left in the pot.
4. Finish the dish. Remove the lid from the Multicooker. Close crisping lid. Select AIR CRISP, set temperature to 375°F, and set time to 15 minutes. Check after 10 minutes, cooking for an additional 5 minutes if dish needs more browning.
Cut the limes, heat the beans put the hot rice into a serving bowl.
Set the Lamb aside. Ladle a generous amount of sauce over it.
Heat up 3-4 corn tortillas.
Put the lamb mixture onto a soft warm corn tortilla, sprinkle on cilantro, then squeeze with lime juice.
Serve and Enjoy

Pulled BBQ Beef Sandwiches
PREP: 10 MINUTES • PRESSURE: 35 MINUTES • AIR CRISP: 15 MINUTES • TOTAL: 60 MINUTES • PRESSURE LEVEL: HIGH • RELEASE: NORMAL
SERVES 2-4

Ingredients

2 pounds – Beef of choice
2 cps – Water
4 cps – Finely shredded Cabbage (the secret ingredient and you'll never know it's in there.)
1/2 cup – Of your favorite BBQ Sauce
1 cup – Ketchup
1/3 cup – Worcestershire Sauce
1 tblsp – Horse Radish
1 tblsp – mustard

Directions

1. Preparing the Ingredients. Add and stir in ingredients to your Multicooker.
2. High pressure for 35 minutes. Lock the lid on the Multicooker and then cook for 35 minutes. To get 35-minutes cook time, press "Pressure" button and adjust the time.
3. Pressure Release. Use natural release method.
4. Finish the dish. Remove the lid from the Multicooker. Close crisping lid. Select AIR CRISP, set temperature to 390°F, and set time to 15 minutes. Check after 10 minutes, cooking for an additional 5 minutes if dish needs more browning.
5. Set the beef aside. Set the Multicooker to a "Sauté" mode, Sauté the sauce until it reaches the desired consistency. Serve and Enjoy.

Air Fryer Burgers

PREP: 5 MINUTES • COOK TIME: 10 MINUTES • TOTAL: 15 MINUTES
SERVES: 4

Ingredients

- 1 pound lean ground beef
- 1 tsp. dried parsley
- ½ tsp. dried oregano
- ½ tsp. pepper
- ½ tsp. salt
- ½ tsp. onion powder
- ½ tsp. garlic powder
- Few drops of liquid smoke
- 1 tsp. Worcestershire sauce

Directions:

1. Preparing the Ingredients. Ensure your Crisplid-Pot is preheated to 350 degrees.

Mix all seasonings together till combined.

Place beef in a bowl and add seasonings. Mix well, but do not overmix.

Make 4 patties from the mixture and using your thumb, making an indent in the center of each patty.

Add patties to Crisplid-Pot basket.

2. Air Frying. Set temperature to 350°F, and set time to 10 minutes, and cook 10 minutes. No need to turn.

PER SERVING: CALORIES: 148; FAT: 5G; PROTEIN:24G; SUGAR:1G

Lamb And Eggplant Pasta Casserole

PREP: 10 MINUTES • PRESSURE: 8 MINUTES • BROIL: 5 MINUTES • TOTAL: 18 MINUTES • PRESSURE LEVEL: HIGH • RELEASE: QUICK
SERVES 4

Ingredients

2 tablespoons olive oil
1 medium red onion, chopped
1 tablespoon minced garlic
1½ pounds lean ground lamb
One small eggplant (about ¾ pound), stemmed and diced
¾ cup dry red wine, such as Syrah
2¼ cups chicken broth
½ cup canned tomato paste
1 teaspoon ground cinnamon
½ tablespoon dried oregano
½ teaspoon dried dill
½ teaspoon salt
½ teaspoon ground black pepper
8 ounces dried spiral-shaped pasta, such as rotini

Directions
1.   Preparing the Ingredients. Heat the oil in the Multicooker turned to the "Sauté" function. Add the onion and cook, often stirring, until softened, about 4 minutes. Add the garlic and cook until aromatic, less than 1 minute.
Crumble in the ground lamb; cook, stirring occasionally until it has lost its raw color, about 5 minutes. Add the eggplant and cook for 1 minute, often stirring, to soften a bit. Pour in the red wine and scrape up any browned bits in the pot as it comes to a simmer.
Stir in the broth, tomato paste, cinnamon, oregano, dill, salt, and pepper until everything is coated in the tomato sauce. Stir in the pasta until coated.
2.   High pressure for 8 minutes. Lock the lid on the Multicooker and then cook for 8 minutes. To get 8-minutes cook time, press "Pressure" button and use the Time Adjustment button to adjust the cook time to 8 minutes.
3.   Pressure Release. Use the quick-release method.

4. Remove the lid from the Multicooker. Close crisping lid. Select BROIL, and set time to 5 minutes. Cooking for an additional 4 minutes if dish needs more browning.

Unlock and open the pot. Stir well before serving.

Lamb Shanks Provençal

PREP: 10 MINUTES • PRESSURE: 40 MINUTES • AIR CRISP: 18 MINUTES • TOTAL: 68 MINUTES • PRESSURE LEVEL: HIGH • RELEASE: NATURAL
SERVES 6

Ingredients

2 large (12-ounce) lamb shanks
1 teaspoon kosher salt, plus additional for seasoning
Freshly ground black pepper
1 tablespoon olive oil
1 cup sliced onion
2 garlic cloves, finely minced
2 medium plum tomatoes, coarsely chopped, or ½ cup diced canned tomatoes, drained
½ cup dry white wine or dry white vermouth
1 cup Chicken Stock or low-sodium broth
1 bay leaf
1 lemon, sliced very thin
⅓ cup pitted Kalamata olives
2 tablespoons coarsely chopped fresh parsley

Directions

1. Preparing the Ingredients. Sprinkle the lamb shanks with 1 teaspoon of kosher salt and several grinds of pepper. The longer ahead of the cooking time you can do this, the better. Cover and let sit for 20 minutes to 2 hours at room temperature or refrigerate for up to 24 hours.

Heat the vegetable oil in the Multicooker using the "Sauté" function, until the oil is shimmering and flows like water. Add the lamb shanks, and brown on all sides, about 6 minutes total. Remove them to a plate. Add the onion and garlic, and sprinkle with a pinch or two of kosher salt. Cook, stirring, for about 3 minutes, or until the onions just begin to brown. Add the tomatoes, and cook until most of their liquid evaporates.

Add the white wine, and stir, scraping up the browned bits from the bottom of the cooker.

Cook for 2 to 3 minutes, or until the wine reduces by about half; then add the Chicken Stock and bay leaf. Return the lamb shanks to the cooker, and place the lemon slices over them.

2. High pressure for 40 minutes. Lock the lid on the Multicooker and then cook for 40 minutes. To get 40-minutes cook time, press "Pressure" button and adjust the time.

3. Pressure Release. After cooking, use the natural method to release pressure.

4. Finish the dish. Remove the lid from the Multicooker. Close crisping lid. Select AIR CRISP, set temperature to 375°F, and set time to 18 minutes. Check after 10 minutes, cooking for an additional 8 minutes if dish needs more browning.

Transfer the lamb to a cutting board or plate, and tent it with aluminum foil. Strain the sauce into a fat separator, and let it rest until the fat rises to the surface.

If you don't have a fat separator, let the sauce sit for a few minutes, then spoon or blot off any excess fat from the top and discard. Pour the defatted sauce back into the cooker along with the strained vegetables. If you want a thicker sauce, simmer the liquid for about 5 minutes, or until it reaches the desired consistency.

Stir in the olives and parsley. Place the shanks in shallow bowls, pour the sauce and vegetables over the lamb, and serve.

Lamb shanks benefit from salting in advance, which makes them much more flavorful and helps them brown beautifully. If you have the time, salt them up to 24 hours in advance. Place them on a tray and refrigerate, covered loosely with foil.

Lamb Shanks With Pancetta

PREP: 15 MINUTES • PRESSURE: 60 MINUTES • AIR CRISP: 18 MINUTES • TOTAL: 75 MINUTES • PRESSURE LEVEL: HIGH • RELEASE: NATURAL
SERVES 4

Ingredients
2 tablespoons olive oil
One 6-ounce pancetta chunk, chopped
Four 12-ounce lamb shanks
1 small yellow onion, chopped
One 28-ounce can diced tomatoes, drained (about 3½ cups)
1 ounce dried mushrooms, preferably porcini, crumbled
3 tablespoons packed celery leaves, minced
2 tablespoons minced chives
2 cups dry, light white wine, such as Sauvignon Blanc
2 tablespoons all-purpose flour
½ teaspoon ground black pepper

Directions

1.   Preparing the Ingredients. Heat the oil in the Multicooker, turned to the "sauté" function. Add the pancetta and brown well, about 6 minutes, stirring often. Use a slotted spoon to transfer the pancetta to a large bowl.
Add two of the shanks to the cooker; brown on all sides, turning occasionally, about 8 minutes. Transfer them to the bowl and repeat with the remaining shanks.
Add the onion to the pot; cook, often stirring, until softened, about 4 minutes. Stir in the tomatoes, dried mushroom

crumbles, celery leaves, and chives. Cook until bubbling, about minutes, stirring often.

Whisk the wine, flour, and pepper in a medium bowl until the flour dissolves; stir this mixture into the sauce in the pot. Cook until thickened and bubbling, about 1 minute.

Return the shanks, pancetta, and their juices to the cooker.

2. High pressure for 60 minutes. Close the lid and the pressure valve and then cook for 60 minutes. To get 60-minutes cook time, press "Pressure" button and use the Time Adjustment button to adjust the cook time to 60 minutes.

Turn off the Multicooker or unplug it, so it doesn't jump to its keep-warm setting.

3. Pressure Release. Let its pressure return to normal naturally, 20 to 30 minutes.

4. Finish the dish. Remove the lid from the Multicooker. Close crisping lid. Select AIR CRISP, set temperature to 375°F, and set time to 18 minutes. Check after 10 minutes, cooking for an additional 8 minutes if dish needs more browning.

Transfer a shank to each serving bowl. Skim any surface fat from the sauce with a flatware spoon. Ladle the sauce and vegetables over the lamb shanks.

Seafood

Pasta with Tuna and Capers

PREP: 2 MINUTES • PRESSURE: 3 MINUTES • TOTAL: 5 MINUTES • PRESSURE LEVEL: HIGH • RELEASE: QUICK
SERVES 2-4

Ingredients

1 tablespoon olive oil
1 garlic clove
3 anchovies
2 cups tomato puree
1½ teaspoons salt
16 oz. (500g) fusilli pasta
2 5.5oz (160g) cans Tuna packed in olive oil water to cover
2 tablespoons capers

Directions

1. Preparing the Ingredients. In the pre-heated Multicooker on "Sauté" mode, add the oil, garlic and anchovies. Sauté until the anchovies begin to disintegrate and the garlic cloves are just starting to turn golden.

Add the tomato puree and salt and mix together.

Pour in the uncooked pasta, and the contents of one tuna can (5 oz.) mixing to coat the dry pasta evenly.

Flatten the pasta in an even layer and pour in just enough water to cover.

2. High pressure for 3 minutes. Lock the lid on the Multicooker and then cook for 3 minutes. To get 3-minutes cook time, press "Pressure" button and use the Time Adjustment button to adjust the cook time to 3 minutes.

3. Pressure Release. When time is up, open the cooker by releasing the pressure.

4. Finish the dish. Mix in the last 5oz of tuna. Close CRISPING LID and select Broil, set time to 7 minutes. Sprinkle with capers before serving.

Enjoy

Shrimp And Tomatillo Casserole

PREP: 10 MINUTES • PRESSURE: 9 MINUTES • BROIL: 5 MINUTES • TOTAL: 30 MINUTES • PRESSURE LEVEL: HIGH • RELEASE: QUICK
SERVES 4

Ingredients
2 tablespoons olive oil
1 medium yellow onion, chopped
1 small fresh jalapeño chile, stemmed, seeded, and minced
2 teaspoons minced garlic
1½ pounds fresh tomatillos, husked and chopped
½ cup bottled clam juice
2 tablespoons fresh lime juice
1½ pounds medium shrimp (about 30 per pound), peeled and deveined
¼ cup loosely packed fresh cilantro leaves, chopped
1 cup shredded Monterey jack cheese (about 4 ounces)

Directions
1.   Preparing the Ingredients. Heat the oil in the Multicooker turned to the "Browning" function. Add the onion and cook, often stirring, until translucent, about 3 minutes.
Add the jalapeño and garlic; cook until aromatic, stirring all the while, less than a minute.
Stir in the tomatillos, clam juice, and lime juice.
2.   High pressure for 9 minutes. Lock the lid on the Multicooker and then cook for 9 minutes. To get 9-minutes cook time, press "Pressure" button and use the Time Adjustment button to adjust the cook time to 9 minutes.
3.   Pressure Release Use the quick-release method.
4.   Finish the dish. Unlock and open the pot. Turn the Multicooker to its "Sauté" function. Stir in the shrimp and cilantro; cook for 2 minutes, stirring frequently. Sprinkle the cheese over the top of the casserole. Close CRISPING LID and

select Broil, set time to 5 minutes. Perss Start/Stop button to begin.
Serve and enjoy.

Fish Filets

PREP: 5 MINUTES • PRESSURE: 5 MINUTES • BROIL: 5 MINUTES • TOTAL: 15 MINUTES • PRESSURE LEVEL: LOW • RELEASE: NORMAL
SERVES 2

Ingredients
4 White Fish fillets (any white fish)
1 lb. (500g) Cherry Tomatoes, halved
1 cup Black salt-cured Olives (Taggiesche, French or Kalamata)
2 Tbsp. Pickled Capers
1 bunch of fresh Thyme Olive Oil
1 clove of garlic, pressed
Salt and pepper to taste

Directions
1.   Preparing the Ingredients. Prepare the base of the Multicooker with 1½ to 2 cups of water and trivet or steamer basket.
Line the bottom of the heat-proof bowl with cherry tomato halves (to keep the fish filet from sticking), add Thyme (reserve a few sprigs for garnish).
Place the fish fillets over the cherry tomatoes, sprinkle with remaining tomatoes, crushed garlic, a dash of olive oil and a pinch of salt.
Insert the dish in the Multicooker - if your heat proof dish does not have handles construct them by making a long aluminum sling.

2. High pressure for 5 minutes. Lock the lid on the Multicooker and then cook for 5 minutes. To get 5-minutes cook time, press "Pressure" button and then adjust the time.
3. Pressure Release. Perform a quick release to release the cooker's pressure.
4. Finish the dish. Close crisping lid and select Broil, set time to 7 minutes.

Distribute fish into individual plates, top with cherry tomatoes, and sprinkle with olives, capers, fresh Thyme, a crackle of pepper and a little swirl of fresh olive oil.

Per Serving Calories: 278.2; Fat: 5.8g; Carbohydrates: 18.8g; Sodium: 1056.8mg; Fiber: 2.5g; Protien: 25.6g

Mediterranean Tuna Noodle Delight

PREP: 6 MINUTES • PRESSURE: 10 MINUTES • BROIL: 7 MINUTES • TOTAL: 23 MINUTES • PRESSURE LEVEL: HIGH • RELEASE: NATURAL
SERVES 2

Ingredients
1 Tablespoon of Oil
½ cup of chopped red onion
8 ounces of dry wide egg noodles (uncooked)
1 can (14 ounces) diced tomatoes with basil, garlic and oregano(undrained) or any kind you have on hand.
1-1/4 cups of water
¼ teaspoon of salt
1/8 teaspoon of pepper
1 can of tuna fish in water, drained
1 jar (7.5 oz.) marinated artichoke hearts, drained with saving the liquid, then chop it up
Crumpled feta cheese

Fresh chopped parsley or dried

Directions
1. Preparing the Ingredients. Sauté the red onion for about 2 minutes.
Add the dry noodles, tomatoes, water, salt and pepper.
2. High pressure for 10 minutes. Lock the lid on the Multicooker and then cook for 10 minutes. To get 10-minutes cook time, press "Pressure" button and adjust the time.
3. Pressure Release. Release the pressure using natural release method.
Turn off the warm setting.
Add tuna, artichokes and your reserved liquid from the artichokes and sauté on normal while stirring for about 4 more minutes till hot, top with a feta cheese to your liking.
4. Close crisping lid and select Broil, set time to 7 minutes. Press Start/Stop button.
Serve.

Per Serving Calories: 258.3; Fat: 5.8g; Carbohydrates: 15.8g; Sugar: 0.2g; Sodium: 1146.8mg; Fiber: 2.5g; Protien: 29.6g

Beer Potato Fish

PREP: 15 MINUTES • PRESSURE: 40 MINUTES • BROIL: 5 MINUTES • TOTAL: 60 MINUTES • PRESSURE LEVEL: LOW • RELEASE: NATURAL
SERVES 6

Ingredients
1 pound fish fillet
4 medium size potatoes, peeled and diced
1 cup beer

1 red pepper sliced
1 tablespoon oil
1 tablespoon oyster flavored sauce
1 tablespoon rock candy
1 teaspoon salt

Directions
1. Preparing the Ingredients. Put all ingredients into your Multicooker.
2. High pressure for 40 minutes. Lock the lid on the Multicooker and then cook for 40 minutes. To get 40-minutes cook time, press "Pressure" button and use the Time Adjustment button to adjust the cook time to 40 minutes.
3. Pressure Release. Release the pressure using natural release method.
4. Finish the dish. Close the crisping lid. Select BROIL, and set the time to 5 minutes. Select START/STOP to begin. Cook until top is browned.
Then that is it! Simple, fast, delicious, retaining flavour and nutrition, consistent results all the time.
Serve and Enjoy!

Per Serving Calories: 250.3; Fat: 4.8g; Sodium: 1146.8mg; Fiber: 2.5g; Protien: 25.6g

Sweet And Savory Breaded Shrimp
PREP: 5 MINUTES • COOK TIME: 20 MINUTES • TOTAL: 25 MINUTES
SERVES: 2

Ingredients
½ pound of fresh shrimp, peeled from their shells and rinsed

2 raw eggs
½ cup of breadcrumbs (we like Panko, but any brand or home recipe will do)
½ white onion, peeled and rinsed and finely chopped
1 teaspoon of ginger-garlic paste
½ teaspoon of turmeric powder
½ teaspoon of red chili powder
½ teaspoon of cumin powder
½ teaspoon of black pepper powder
½ teaspoon of dry mango powder
Pinch of salt

Directions:
1   Preparing the Ingredients. Cover the basket of the Crisplid-Pot with a lining of tin foil, leaving the edges uncovered to allow air to circulate through the basket.

Preheat the Crisplid-Pot to 350 degrees.

In a large mixing bowl, beat the eggs until fluffy and until the yolks and whites are fully combined.

Dunk all the shrimp in the egg mixture, fully submerging.

In a separate mixing bowl, combine the bread crumbs with all the dry ingredients until evenly blended.

One by one, coat the egg-covered shrimp in the mixed dry ingredients so that fully covered, and place on the foil-lined air-fryer basket.

2   Air Frying. Set the air-fryer timer to 20 minutes.

Halfway through the cooking time, shake the handle of the air-fryer so that the breaded shrimp jostles inside and fry-coverage is even.

After 20 minutes, when the fryer shuts off, the shrimp will be perfectly cooked and their breaded crust golden-brown and delicious! Using tongs, remove from the Crisplid-Pot and set on a serving dish to cool.

Coconut Shrimp

PREP: 15 MINUTES • COOK TIME: 5 MINUTES • TOTAL: 20 MINUTES
SERVES: 4

Ingredients

- 1 (8-ounce) can crushed pineapple
- ½ cup sour cream
- ¼ cup pineapple preserves
- 2 egg whites
- ⅔ cup cornstarch
- ⅔ cup sweetened coconut
- 1 cup panko bread crumbs
- 1 pound uncooked large shrimp, thawed if frozen, deveined and shelled
- Olive oil for misting

Directions:

1. Preparing the Ingredients. Drain the crushed pineapple well, reserving the juice. In a small bowl, combine the pineapple, sour cream, and preserves, and mix well. Set aside. In a shallow bowl, beat the egg whites with 2 tablespoons of the reserved pineapple liquid. Place the cornstarch on a plate. Combine the coconut and bread crumbs on another plate. Dip the shrimp into the cornstarch, shake it off, then dip into the egg white mixture and finally into the coconut mixture. Place the shrimp in the Crisplid-Pot basket and mist with oil.

2. Air Frying. Air-fry for 5 to 7 minutes or until the shrimp are crisp and golden brown.

PER SERVING: CALORIES: 524; FAT: 14G; PROTEIN:33G; FIBER:4G

Cilantro-Lime Fried Shrimp

PREP: 10 MINUTES • COOK TIME: 10 MINUTES • TOTAL: 20 MINUTES
SERVES: 4

Ingredients
1 pound raw shrimp, peeled and deveined with tails on or off (see Prep tip)
½ cup chopped fresh cilantro
Juice of 1 lime
1 egg
½ cup all-purpose flour
¾ cup bread crumbs
Salt
Pepper
Cooking oil
½ cup cocktail sauce (optional)

Directions:

1   Preparing the Ingredients. Place the shrimp in a plastic bag and add the cilantro and lime juice. Seal the bag. Shake to combine. Marinate in the refrigerator for 30 minutes.
In a small bowl, beat the egg. In another small bowl, place the flour. Place the bread crumbs in a third small bowl, and season with salt and pepper to taste.
Spray the Crisplid-Pot basket with cooking oil.
Remove the shrimp from the plastic bag. Dip each in the flour, then the egg, and then the bread crumbs.

2   Air Frying. Place the shrimp in the Crisplid-Pot. It is okay to stack them. Spray the shrimp with cooking oil. Cook for 4 minutes.

Open the Crisplid-Pot and flip the shrimp. I recommend flipping individually instead of shaking to keep the breading intact. Cook for an additional 4 minutes, or until crisp.
Cool before serving. Serve with cocktail sauce if desired.

PER SERVING: CALORIES: 254; FAT:4G; PROTEIN:29G; FIBER:1G

Lemony Tuna

PREP: 10 MINUTES • COOK TIME: 10 MINUTES • TOTAL: 20 MINUTES
SERVES: 4

Ingredients
2 (6-ounce) cans water packed plain tuna
  2 teaspoons Dijon mustard
  ½ cup breadcrumbs
  1 tablespoon fresh lime juice
  2 tablespoons fresh parsley, chopped
  1 egg
  3 tablespoons canola oil
  Salt and freshly ground black pepper, to taste

Directions:
1   Preparing the Ingredients. Drain most of the liquid from the canned tuna.
In a bowl, add the fish, mustard, crumbs, citrus juice, parsley, and hot sauce and mix till well combined. Add a little canola oil if it seems too dry. Add egg, salt and stir to combine. Make the patties from tuna mixture. Refrigerate the tuna patties for about 2 hours.
2   Air Frying. Preheat the Crisplid-Pot to 355 degrees F. Cook for about 10-12 minutes.

Grilled Soy Salmon Fillets

PREP: 5 MINUTES • COOK TIME: 8 MINUTES • TOTAL: 13 MINUTES
SERVES: 4

Ingredients
- 4 salmon fillets
- 1/4 teaspoon ground black pepper
- 1/2 teaspoon cayenne pepper
- 1/2 teaspoon salt
- 1 teaspoon onion powder
- 1 tablespoon fresh lemon juice
- 1/2 cup soy sauce
- 1/2 cup water
- 1 tablespoon honey
- 2 tablespoons extra-virgin olive oil

Directions:
1. Preparing the Ingredients. Firstly, pat the salmon fillets dry using kitchen towels. Season the salmon with black pepper, cayenne pepper, salt, and onion powder.

To make the marinade, combine together the lemon juice, soy sauce, water, honey, and olive oil. Marinate the salmon for at least 2 hours in your refrigerator.

Arrange the fish fillets on a grill basket in your Crisplid-Pot.

2. Air Frying. Bake at 330 degrees for 8 to 9 minutes, or until salmon fillets are easily flaked with a fork.

Work with batches and serve warm.

Scallops and Spring Veggies

PREP: 10 MINUTES • COOK TIME: 8 MINUTES • TOTAL: 18 MINUTES
SERVES: 4

Ingredients
½ pound asparagus ends trimmed, cut into 2-inch pieces
1 cup sugar snap peas
1 pound sea scallops
1 tablespoon lemon juice
2 teaspoons olive oil
½ teaspoon dried thyme
Pinch salt
Freshly ground black pepper

Directions:
1   Preparing the Ingredients. Place the asparagus and sugar snap peas in the Crisplid-Pot basket.
2   Air Frying. Cook for 2 to 3 minutes or until the vegetables are just starting to get tender.
Meanwhile, check the scallops for a small muscle attached to the side, and pull it off and discard.
In a medium bowl, toss the scallops with the lemon juice, olive oil, thyme, salt, and pepper. Place into the Crisplid-Pot basket on top of the vegetables.
3   Air Frying. Steam for 5 to 7 minutes, tossing the basket once during cooking time, until the scallops are just firm when tested with your finger and are opaque in the center, and the vegetables are tender. Serve immediately.

PER SERVING: CALORIES: 162; CARBS:10G; FAT: 4G; PROTEIN:22G; FIBER:3G

Fried Calamari

PREP: 8 MINUTES • COOK TIME: 7 MINUTES • TOTAL: 15 MINUTES
SERVES: 6-8

Ingredients

- ½ tsp. salt
- ½ tsp. Old Bay seasoning
- 1/3 C. plain cornmeal
- ½ C. semolina flour
- ½ C. almond flour
- 5-6 C. olive oil
- 1 ½ pounds baby squid

Directions:

1. Preparing the Ingredients. Rinse squid in cold water and slice tentacles, keeping just ¼-inch of the hood in one piece. Combine 1-2 pinches of pepper, salt, Old Bay seasoning, cornmeal, and both flours together. Dredge squid pieces into flour mixture and place into the Crisplid-Pot.
2. Air Frying. Spray liberally with olive oil. Cook 15 minutes at 345 degrees till coating turns a golden brown.

PER SERVING: CALORIES: 211; CARBS:55; FAT: 6G; PROTEIN:21G; SUGAR:1G

Soy and Ginger Shrimp

PREP: 8 MINUTES • COOK TIME: 10 MINUTES • TOTAL: 15 MINUTES

SERVES: 4

Ingredients
- 2 tablespoons olive oil
- 2 tablespoons scallions, finely chopped
- 2 cloves garlic, chopped
- 1 teaspoon fresh ginger, grated
- 1 tablespoon dry white wine
- 1 tablespoon balsamic vinegar
- 1/4 cup soy sauce
- 1 tablespoon sugar
- 1 pound shrimp
- Salt and ground black pepper, to taste

Directions:

1 Preparing the Ingredients. To make the marinade, warm the oil in a saucepan; cook all ingredients, except the shrimp, salt, and black pepper. Now, let it cool.

Marinate the shrimp, covered, at least an hour, in the refrigerator.

2 Air Frying. After that, bake the shrimp at 350 degrees F for 8 to 10 minutes (depending on the size), turning once or twice. Season prepared shrimp with salt and black pepper and serve right away.

Crispy Cheesy Fish Fingers

PREP: 10 MINUTES • COOK TIME: 20 MINUTES • TOTAL: 30 MINUTES
SERVES: 4

Ingredients
- Large codfish filet, approximately 6-8 ounces, fresh or frozen and thawed, cut into 1 ½-inch strips
- 2 raw eggs

½ cup of breadcrumbs (we like Panko, but any brand or home recipe will do)
2 tablespoons of shredded or powdered parmesan cheese
1 tablespoons of shredded cheddar cheese
Pinch of salt and pepper

Directions:

1   Preparing the Ingredients. Cover the basket of the Crisplid-Pot with a lining of tin foil, leaving the edges uncovered to allow air to circulate through the basket.

Preheat the Crisplid-Pot to 350 degrees.

In a large mixing bowl, beat the eggs until fluffy and until the yolks and whites are fully combined.

Dunk all the fish strips in the beaten eggs, fully submerging.

In a separate mixing bowl, combine the bread crumbs with the parmesan, cheddar, and salt and pepper, until evenly mixed.

One by one, coat the egg-covered fish strips in the mixed dry ingredients so that they're fully covered, and place on the foil-lined Crisplid-Pot basket.

2   Air Frying. Set the air-fryer timer to 20 minutes.

Halfway through the cooking time, shake the handle of the air-fryer so that the breaded fish jostles inside and fry-coverage is even.

After 20 minutes, when the fryer shuts off, the fish strips will be perfectly cooked and their breaded crust golden-brown and delicious! Using tongs, remove from the Crisplid-Pot and set on a serving dish to cool.

Fish Cakes With Mango Relish
PREP: 5 MINUTES • COOK TIME: 10 MINUTES • TOTAL: 15 MINUTES
SERVES: 4

Ingredients
- 1 lb White Fish Fillets
- 3 Tbsps Ground Coconut
- 1 Ripened Mango
- ½ Tsps Chili Paste
- Tbsps Fresh Parsley
- 1 Green Onion
- 1 Lime
- 1 Tsp Salt
- 1 Egg

Directions:

1. Preparing the Ingredients. To make the relish, peel and dice the mango into cubes. Combine with a half teaspoon of chili paste, a tablespoon of parsley, and the zest and juice of half a lime.

In a food processor, pulse the fish until it forms a smooth texture. Place into a bowl and add the salt, egg, chopped green onion, parsley, two tablespoons of the coconut, and the remainder of the chili paste and lime zest and juice. Combine well

Portion the mixture into 10 equal balls and flatten them into small patties. Pour the reserved tablespoon of coconut onto a dish and roll the patties over to coat.

Preheat the Crisplid-Pot to 390 degrees

2. Air Frying. Place the fish cakes into the Crisplid-Pot and cook for 8 minutes. They should be crisp and lightly browned when ready

Serve hot with mango relish

Firecracker Shrimp

PREP: 10 MINUTES • COOK TIME: 8 MINUTES • TOTAL: 18 MINUTES
SERVES: 4

Ingredients

For the shrimp
- 1 pound raw shrimp, peeled and deveined
- Salt
- Pepper
- 1 egg
- ½ cup all-purpose flour
- ¾ cup panko bread crumbs
- Cooking oil

For the firecracker sauce
- ⅓ cup sour cream
- 2 tablespoons Sriracha
- ¼ cup sweet chili sauce

Directions:

1. **Preparing the Ingredients.** Season the shrimp with salt and pepper to taste. In a small bowl, beat the egg. In another small bowl, place the flour. In a third small bowl, add the panko bread crumbs.

    Spray the Crisplid-Pot basket with cooking oil. Dip the shrimp in the flour, then the egg, and then the bread crumbs. Place the shrimp in the Crisplid-Pot basket. It is okay to stack them. Spray the shrimp with cooking oil.

2. **Air Frying.** Cook for 4 minutes. Open the Crisplid-Pot and flip the shrimp. I recommend flipping individually instead of shaking to keep the breading intact. Cook for an additional 4 minutes or until crisp.

While the shrimp is cooking, make the firecracker sauce: In a small bowl, combine the sour cream, Sriracha, and sweet chili sauce. Mix well. Serve with the shrimp.

PER SERVING: CALORIES: 266; CARBS:23g; FAT:6G; PROTEIN:27G; FIBER:1G

Sesame Seeds Coated Fish

PREP: 10 MINUTES • COOK TIME: 8 MINUTES • TOTAL: 18 MINUTES
SERVES:5

Ingredients
- 3 tablespoons plain flour
- 2 eggs
- ½ cup sesame seeds, toasted
- ½ cup breadcrumbs
- 1/8 teaspoon dried rosemary, crushed
- Pinch of salt
- Pinch of black pepper
- 3 tablespoons olive oil
- 5 frozen fish fillets (white fish of your choice)

Directions:

1. Preparing the Ingredients. In a shallow dish, place flour. In a second shallow dish, beat the eggs. In a third shallow dish, add remaining ingredients except fish fillets and mix till a crumbly mixture forms.

Coat the fillets with flour and shake off the excess flour.
Next, dip the fillets in the egg.
Then coat the fillets with sesame seeds mixture generously.
Preheat the Crisplid-Pot to 390 degrees F.

2. Air Frying. Line an Crisplid-Pot basket with a piece of foil. Arrange the fillets into prepared basket.

Cook for about 14 minutes, flipping once after 10 minutes.

Crispy Paprika Fish Fillets

PREP: 5 MINUTES • COOK TIME: 15 MINUTES • TOTAL: 20 MINUTES
SERVES: 4

Ingredients
- 1/2 cup seasoned breadcrumbs
- 1 tablespoon balsamic vinegar
- 1/2 teaspoon seasoned salt
- 1 teaspoon paprika
- 1/2 teaspoon ground black pepper
- 1 teaspoon celery seed
- 2 fish fillets, halved
- 1 egg, beaten

Directions:
1   Preparing the Ingredients. Add the breadcrumbs, vinegar, salt, paprika, ground black pepper, and celery seeds to your food processor. Process for about 30 seconds.
Coat the fish fillets with the beaten egg; then, coat them with the breadcrumbs mixture.
2   Air Frying. Cook at 350 degrees F for about 15 minutes.

Parmesan Shrimp

PREP: 5 MINUTES • COOK TIME: 10 MINUTES • TOTAL: 15 MINUTES
SERVES: 4

Ingredients
- 2 tbsp. olive oil
- 1 tsp. onion powder
- 1 tsp. basil
- ½ tsp. oregano
- 1 tsp. pepper

2/3 C. grated parmesan cheese
4 minced garlic cloves
pounds of jumbo cooked shrimp (peeled/deveined)

Directions:
1   Preparing the Ingredients. Mix all seasonings together and gently toss shrimp with the mixture.
2   Air Frying. Spray olive oil into the Crisplid-Pot basket and add seasoned shrimp.
Cook 8-10 minutes at 350 degrees.
Squeeze lemon juice over shrimp right before devouring!

-
  PER SERVING: CALORIES: 351; FAT:11G; PROTEIN:19G; SUGAR:1G

-

Fish and Chips

PREP: 10 MINUTES • COOK TIME: 20 MINUTES • TOTAL: 30 MINUTES
SERVES: 4

Ingredients
4 (4-ounce) fish fillets
Pinch salt
Freshly ground black pepper
½ teaspoon dried thyme
1 egg white
¾ cup crushed potato chips
2 tablespoons olive oil, divided
1   russet potatoes, peeled and cut into strips

Directions:

1   Preparing the Ingredients. Pat the fish fillets dry and sprinkle with salt, pepper, and thyme. Set aside.

In a shallow bowl, beat the egg white until foamy. In another bowl, combine the potato chips and 1 tablespoon of olive oil and mix until combined.

Dip the fish fillets into the egg white, then into the crushed potato chip mixture to coat.

Toss the fresh potato strips with the remaining 1 tablespoon olive oil.

2   Air Frying. Use your separator to divide the Crisplid-Pot basket in half, then fry the chips and fish. The chips will take about 20 minutes; the fish will take about 10 to 12 minutes to cook.

PER SERVING: CALORIES: 374; FAT:16G; PROTEIN:30G; FIBER:4G

Sweet Recipes

Fried Peaches

PREP: 2 HOURS 10 MINUTES • COOK TIME: 15 MINUTES • TOTAL: 15 MINUTES
SERVES: 4

Ingredients
- 4 ripe peaches (1/2 a peach = 1 serving)
- 1 1/2 cups flour
- Salt
- 2 egg yolks
- 3/4 cups cold water
- 1 1/2 tablespoons olive oil
- 2 tablespoons brandy
- 4 egg whites
- Cinnamon/sugar mix

Directions:

1. Preparing the Ingredients. Mix flour, egg yolks, and salt in a mixing bowl. Slowly mix in water, then add brandy. Set the mixture aside for 2 hours and go do something for 1 hour 45 minutes.

Boil a large pot of water and cut an X at the bottom of each peach. While the water boils, fill another large bowl with water and ice. Boil each peach for about a minute, then plunge it in the ice bath. Now the peels should basically fall off the peach. Beat the egg whites and mix into the batter mix. Dip each peach in the mix to coat.

2. Air Frying. Cook at 360 degrees for 10 Minutes.

Prepare a plate with cinnamon/sugar mix, roll peaches in the mix and serve.

PER SERVING: CALORIES: 306; FAT:.3G; PROTEIN:10G; FIBER:2.7G

Apple Dumplings

PREP: 10 MINUTES • COOK TIME: 25 MINUTES • TOTAL: 35 MINUTES
SERVES: 4

Ingredients
- 2 tbsp. melted coconut oil
- 2 puff pastry sheets
- 1 tbsp. brown sugar
- 2 tbsp. raisins
- 2 small apples of choice

Directions:

1. Preparing the Ingredients. Ensure your Crisplid-Pot is preheated to 356 degrees.
Core and peel apples and mix with raisins and sugar.
Place a bit of apple mixture into puff pastry sheets and brush sides with melted coconut oil.
2. Air Frying. Place into the Crisplid-Pot. Cook 25 minutes, turning halfway through. Will be golden when done.

PER SERVING: CALORIES: 367; FAT:7G; PROTEIN:2G; SUGAR:5

Easy Donuts

PREP: 5 MINUTES • BAKE: 5 MINUTES • PRESSURE: 5 MINUTES • TOTAL: 10 MINUTES
SERVES 8

Ingredients:
Pinch of allspice

4 tbsp. dark brown sugar
½ - 1 tsp. cinnamon
1/3 C. granulated sweetener
3 tbsp. melted coconut oil
1 can of biscuits

Directions
1. Preparing the ingredients. Preheat the unit by selecting Bake/Roast, setting the temperature to 300°F, and setting the time to 5 minutes. Press Start/Stop to begin.
Mix allspice, sugar, sweetener, and cinnamon together.
Take out biscuits from can and with a circle cookie cutter, cut holes from centers and place into Multicooker.
2. Air Frying the Dish. Close the Crisping Lid. Select Bake/Roast, set the temperature to 350°F, and set the time to 5 minutes. Select Start/Stop to begin. As batches are cooked, use a brush to coat with melted coconut oil and dip each into sugar mixture.
Serve warm!

Cinnamon Rolls

PREP: 15 MINUTES • BAKE: 10 MINUTES • TOTAL: 25 MINUTES
SERVES 8

Ingredients:
1 ½ tbsp. cinnamon
¾ C. brown sugar
¼ C. melted coconut oil
1 pound frozen bread dough, thawed

Glaze:

½ tsp. vanilla
1 ¼ C. powdered erythritol
2 tbsp. softened ghee
4 ounces softened cream cheese

Directions:
1. Preparing the ingredients. Preheat the unit by selecting Bake/Roast, setting the temperature to 300°F, and setting the time to 5 minutes. Press Start/Stop to begin. Lay out bread dough and roll out into a rectangle. Brush melted ghee over dough and leave a 1-inch border along edges.
Mix cinnamon and sweetener together and then sprinkle over dough. Roll dough tightly and slice into 8 pieces. Let sit 1-2 hours to rise. To make the glaze, simply mix ingredients together till smooth.
2. Finish the dish. Once rolls rise, place into the Multicooker. Select Bake/Roast, set the temperature to 350°F, and set the time to 5 minutes. Select Start/Stop to begin.
Serve rolls drizzled in cream cheese glaze. Enjoy!

Raspberry Cream Rol-Ups
PREP: 10 MINUTES • COOK TIME: 25 MINUTES • TOTAL: 35 MINUTES
SERVES: 4

Ingredients
1 cup of fresh raspberries rinsed and patted dry
½ cup of cream cheese softened to room temperature
¼ cup of brown sugar
¼ cup of sweetened condensed milk
1 egg
1 teaspoon of corn starch

6 spring roll wrappers (any brand will do, we like Blue Dragon or Tasty Joy, both available through Target or Walmart, or any large grocery chain)
¼ cup of water

Directions:

1   Preparing the Ingredients. Cover the basket of the Crisplid-Pot with a lining of tin foil, leaving the edges uncovered to allow air to circulate through the basket. Preheat the Crisplid-Pot to 350 degrees.

In a mixing bowl, combine the cream cheese, brown sugar, condensed milk, cornstarch, and egg. Beat or whip thoroughly, until all ingredients are completely mixed and fluffy, thick and stiff.

Spoon even amounts of the creamy filling into each spring roll wrapper, then top each dollop of filling with several raspberries.

Roll up the wraps around the creamy raspberry filling, and seal the seams with a few dabs of water.

Place each roll on the foil-lined Crisplid-Pot basket, seams facing down.

2   Air Frying. Set the Crisplid-Pot timer to 10 minutes. During cooking, shake the handle of the fryer basket to ensure a nice even surface crisp.

After 10 minutes, when the Crisplid-Pot shuts off, the spring rolls should be golden brown and perfect on the outside, while the raspberries and cream filling will have cooked together in a glorious fusion. Remove with tongs and serve hot or cold.

Air Fryer Chocolate Cake

PREP: 5 MINUTES • COOK TIME: 35 MINUTES • TOTAL: 40 MINUTES
SERVES: 8-10

Ingredients
- ½ C. hot water
- 1 tsp. vanilla
- ¼ C. olive oil
- ½ C. almond milk
- 1 egg
- ½ tsp. salt
- ¾ tsp. baking soda
- ¾ tsp. baking powder
- ½ C. unsweetened cocoa powder
- 2 C. almond flour
- 1 C. brown sugar

Directions:

1. Preparing the Ingredients. Preheat your Crisplid-Pot to 356 degrees.

Stir all dry ingredients together. Then stir in wet ingredients. Add hot water last.

The batter will be thin, no worries.

2. Air Frying. Pour cake batter into a pan that fits into the fryer. Cover with foil and poke holes into the foil.

Bake 35 minutes.

Discard foil and then bake another 10 minutes.

PER SERVING: CALORIES: 378; FAT:9G; PROTEIN:4G; SUGAR:5G

Chocolate Donuts
PREP: 5 MINUTES • COOK TIME: 20 MINUTES • TOTAL: 25 MINUTES
SERVES: 8-10

Ingredients
(8-ounce) can jumbo biscuits
Cooking oil
Chocolate sauce, such as Hershey's

Directions:
1. Preparing the Ingredients. Separate the biscuit dough into 8 biscuits and place them on a flat work surface. Use a small circle cookie cutter or a biscuit cutter to cut a hole in the center of each biscuit. You can also cut the holes using a knife.

Spray the Crisplid-Pot basket with cooking oil.

2. Air Frying. Place 4 donuts in the Crisplid-Pot. Do not stack. Spray with cooking oil. Cook for 4 minutes.

Open the Crisplid-Pot and flip the donuts. Cook for an additional 4 minutes.

Remove the cooked donuts from the Crisplid-Pot, then repeat steps 3 and 4 for the remaining 4 donuts.

Drizzle chocolate sauce over the donuts and enjoy while warm.

PER SERVING: CALORIES: 181; FAT:98G; PROTEIN:3G; FIBER:1G

Fried Bananas with Chocolate Sauce
PREP: 10 MINUTES • COOK TIME: 10 MINUTES • TOTAL: 20 MINUTES
SERVES: 2

Ingredients
- 1 large egg
- ¼ cup cornstarch
- ¼ cup plain bread crumbs
- 3 bananas, halved crosswise
- Cooking oil
- Chocolate sauce (see Ingredient tip)

Directions:

1. Preparing the Ingredients. In a small bowl, beat the egg. In another bowl, place the cornstarch. Place the bread crumbs in a third bowl. Dip the bananas in the cornstarch, then the egg, and then the bread crumbs.

Spray the Crisplid-Pot basket with cooking oil. Place the bananas in the basket and spray them with cooking oil.

2. Air Frying. Cook for 5 minutes. Open the Crisplid-Pot and flip the bananas. Cook for an additional 2 minutes. Transfer the bananas to plates.

Drizzle the chocolate sauce over the bananas, and serve.

You can make your own chocolate sauce using 2 tablespoons milk and ¼ cup chocolate chips. Heat a saucepan over medium-high heat. Add the milk and stir for 1 to 2 minutes. Add the chocolate chips. Stir for 2 minutes, or until the chocolate has melted.

PER SERVING: CALORIES: 203; FAT:6G; PROTEIN:3G; FIBER:3G

Apple Hand Pies
PREP: 5 MINUTES • COOK TIME: 8 MINUTES • TOTAL: 13 MINUTES

SERVES: 6

Ingredients
15-ounces no-sugar-added apple pie filling
1 store-bought crust

Directions:
1   Preparing the Ingredients. Lay out pie crust and slice into equal-sized squares.
Place 2 tbsp. filling into each square and seal crust with a fork.
2   Air Frying. Place into the Crisplid-Pot. Cook 8 minutes at 390 degrees until golden in color.

PER SERVING: CALORIES: 278; FAT:10G; PROTEIN:5G; SUGAR:4G

Chocolaty Banana Muffins

PREP: 5 MINUTES • COOK TIME: 25 MINUTES • TOTAL: 35 MINUTES
SERVES: 12

Ingredients
¾ cup whole wheat flour
¾ cup plain flour
¼ cup cocoa powder
¼ teaspoon baking powder
1 teaspoon baking soda
¼ teaspoon salt
2 large bananas, peeled and mashed
1 cup sugar
1/3 cup canola oil
1 egg

½ teaspoon vanilla essence
1 cup mini chocolate chips

Directions:

1   Preparing the Ingredients. In a large bowl, mix together flour, cocoa powder, baking powder, baking soda, and salt.
In another bowl, add bananas, sugar, oil, egg and vanilla extract and beat till well combined.
Slowly, add flour mixture in egg mixture and mix till just combined.
Fold in chocolate chips.
Preheat the Airfryer to 345 degrees F. Grease 12 muffin molds.
2   Air Frying. Transfer the mixture into prepared muffin molds evenly and cook for about 20-25 minutes or till a toothpick inserted in the center comes out clean.
Remove the muffin molds from Crisplid-Pot and keep on wire rack to cool for about 10 minutes. Carefully turn on a wire rack to cool completely before serving.

Blueberry Lemon Muffins

PREP: 5 MINUTES • COOK TIME: 10 MINUTES • TOTAL: 15 MINUTES
SERVES: 12

Ingredients

1 tsp. vanilla
Juice and zest of 1 lemon
2 eggs
1 C. blueberries
½ C. cream
¼ C. avocado oil
½ C. monk fruit

2 ½ C. almond flour

Directions:
1   Preparing the Ingredients. Mix monk fruit and flour together.
In another bowl, mix vanilla, egg, lemon juice, and cream together. Add mixtures together and blend well.
Spoon batter into cupcake holders.
2   Air Frying. Place in the Crisplid-Pot. Bake 10 minutes at 320 degrees, checking at 6 minutes to ensure you don't overbake them.

PER SERVING: CALORIES: 317; FAT:11G; PROTEIN:3G; SUGAR:5G

Sweet Cream Cheese Wontons

PREP: 5 MINUTES • COOK TIME: 5 MINUTES • TOTAL: 10 MINUTES
SERVES: 16

Ingredients
1 egg mixed with a bit of water
Wonton wrappers
½ C. powdered erythritol
8 ounces softened cream cheese
Olive oil

Directions:
1   Preparing the Ingredients. Mix sweetener and cream cheese together.

Lay out 4 wontons at a time and cover with a dish towel to prevent drying out.

Place ½ of a teaspoon of cream cheese mixture into each wrapper.

Dip finger into egg/water mixture and fold diagonally to form a triangle. Seal edges well.

Repeat with remaining ingredients.

2. Air Frying. Place filled wontons into the Crisplid-Pot and cook 5 minutes at 400 degrees, shaking halfway through cooking.

PER SERVING: CALORIES: 303; FAT:3G; PROTEIN:0.5G; SUGAR:4G

Air Fryer Cinnamon Rolls

PREP: 15 MINUTES • COOK TIME: 5 MINUTES • TOTAL: 15 MINUTES
SERVES: 8

Ingredients
- 1 ½ tbsp. cinnamon
- ¾ C. brown sugar
- ¼ C. melted coconut oil
- 1 pound frozen bread dough, thawed

Glaze:
- ½ tsp. vanilla
- 1 ¼ C. powdered erythritol
- 2 tbsp. softened ghee
- 3 ounces softened cream cheese

Directions:

1   Preparing the Ingredients. Lay out bread dough and roll out into a rectangle. Brush melted ghee over dough and leave a 1-inch border along edges.

Mix cinnamon and sweetener together and then sprinkle over the dough.

Roll dough tightly and slice into 8 pieces. Let sit 1-2 hours to rise.

To make the glaze, simply mix ingredients together till smooth.

2   Air Frying. Once rolls rise, place into the Crisplid-Pot and cook 5 minutes at 350 degrees.

Serve rolls drizzled in cream cheese glaze. Enjoy!

PER SERVING: CALORIES: 390; FAT:8G; PROTEIN:1G; SUGAR:7G

Black and White Brownies

PREP: 10 MINUTES • COOK TIME: 20 MINUTES • TOTAL: 30 MINUTES
SERVES: 8

Ingredients
- 1 egg
- ¼ cup brown sugar
- 2 tablespoons white sugar
- 2 tablespoons safflower oil
- 1 teaspoon vanilla
- ¼ cup cocoa powder
- ⅓ cup all-purpose flour
- ¼ cup white chocolate chips
- Nonstick baking spray with flour

Directions:

1   Preparing the Ingredients. In a medium bowl, beat the egg with the brown sugar and white sugar. Beat in the oil and vanilla.

Add the cocoa powder and flour, and stir just until combined. Fold in the white chocolate chips.

Spray a 6-by-6-by-2-inch baking pan with nonstick spray. Spoon the brownie batter into the pan.

2   Air Frying. Bake for 20 minutes or until the brownies are set when lightly touched with a finger. Let cool for 30 minutes before slicing to serve.

PER SERVING: CALORIES: 81; FAT:4G; PROTEIN:1G; FIBER:1G

Baked Apple

PREP: 5 MINUTES • COOK TIME: 20 MINUTES • TOTAL: 25 MINUTES
SERVES: 4

Ingredients
- ¼ C. water
- ¼ tsp. nutmeg
- ¼ tsp. cinnamon
- 1 ½ tsp. melted ghee
- 2 tbsp. raisins
- 2 tbsp. chopped walnuts
- 1 medium apple

Directions:

1   Preparing the Ingredients. Preheat your Crisplid-Pot to 350 degrees.

Slice an apple in half and discard some of the flesh from the center.
Place into frying pan.
Mix remaining ingredients together except water. Spoon mixture to the middle of apple halves.
Pour water overfilled apples.

2   Air Frying. Place pan with apple halves into the Crisplid-Pot, bake 20 minutes.

PER SERVING: CALORIES: 199; FAT:9G; PROTEIN:1G; SUGAR:3G

Cinnamon Fried Bananas

PREP: 5 MINUTES • COOK TIME: 10 MINUTES • TOTAL: 15 MINUTES
SERVES: 2-3

Ingredients
- 1 C. panko breadcrumbs
- 3 tbsp. cinnamon
- ½ C. almond flour
- 3 egg whites
- 8 ripe bananas
- 3 tbsp. vegan coconut oil

Directions:

1   Preparing the Ingredients. Heat coconut oil and add breadcrumbs. Mix around 2-3 minutes until golden. Pour into bowl.
Peel and cut bananas in half. Roll each bananas half into flour, eggs, and crumb mixture.

2   Air Frying. Place into the Crisplid-Pot. Cook 10 minutes at 280 degrees.

A great addition to a healthy banana split!

PER SERVING: CALORIES: 219; FAT:10G; PROTEIN:3G; SUGAR:5G

HERITAGE OF FOOD: A FAMILY GATHERING

To survive, we need to eat. As a result, food has turned into a symbol of loving, nurturing and sharing with one another. Recording, collecting, sharing and remembering the recipes that have been passed to you by your family is a great way to immortalize and honor your family. It is these traditions that carve out your individual personality. You will not just be honoring your family tradition by cooking these recipes, but they will also inspire you to create your own variations, which you can then pass on to your children's.

The recipes are just passed on to everyone, and nobody actually possesses them. I too love sharing recipes. The collection is vibrant and rich as a number of home cooks have offered their inputs to ensure that all of us can cook delicious meals at our home. I am thankful to each one of you who has contributed to this book and has allowed their traditions to pass on and grow with others. You guys are wonderful!

I am also thankful to the cooks who have evaluated all these recipes. You're, as well as, the comments that came from your family members and friends were invaluable.

www.ingramcontent.com/pod-product-compliance
Lightning Source LLC
Chambersburg PA
CBHW072010070526
44583CB00015B/1413